Beauty: Pure + Simple

A HOLISTIC GUIDE TO NATURAL BEAUTY

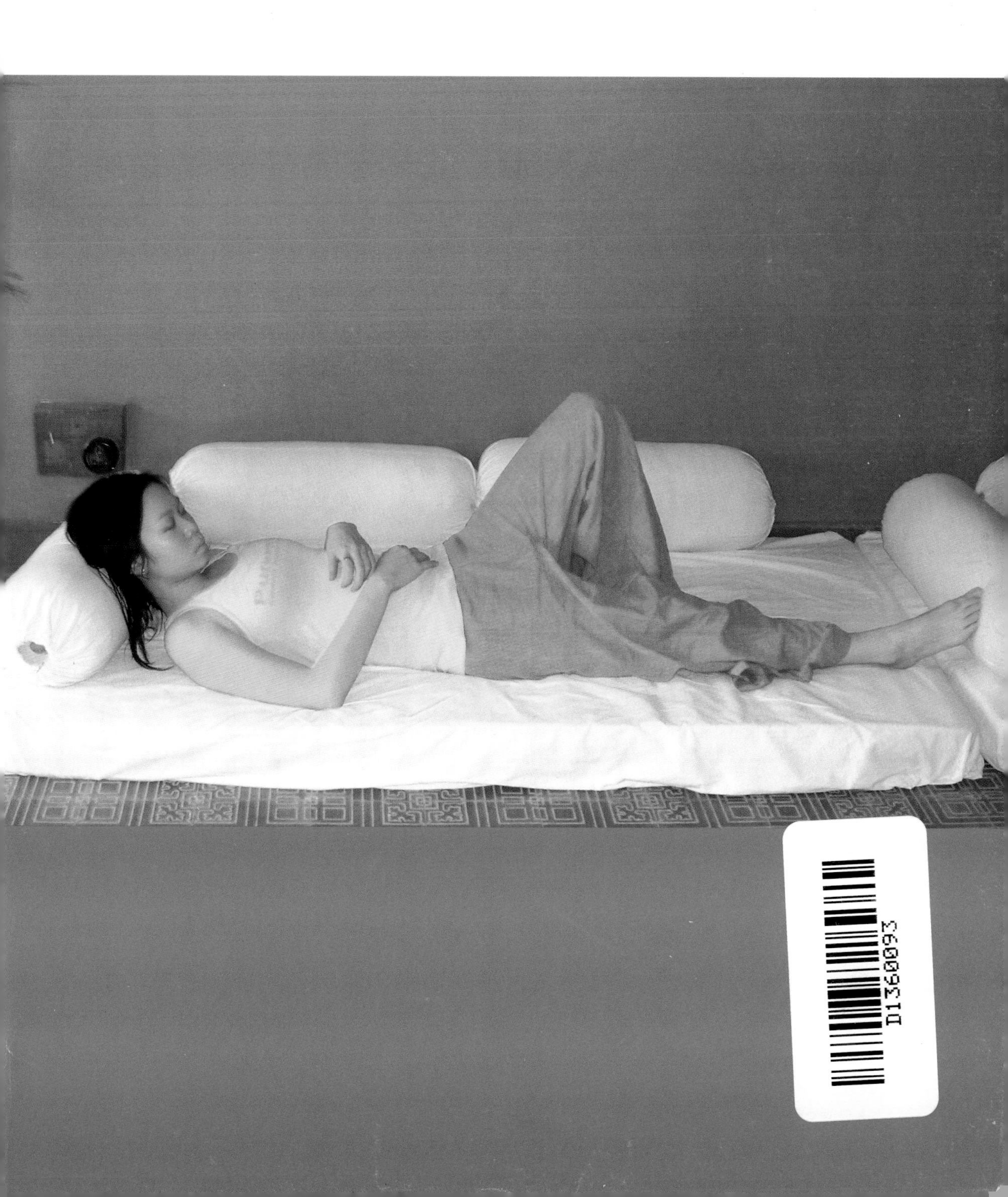

Acknowledgements

As with all successes in my life, I have a team of people to thank for their contributions and support. I would like to thank:

My mother Jean who has provided me with so much opportunity. Your Vata energy has kept the momentum and movement of this project going.

Dr. Lad, Dr. Ranade, Dr. Lele, and Dr. Yan for teaching and inspiring me to transform my view of health, skin and love.

Dr. Lewis who has encouraged me so much and always emphasized the importance of discipline. I especially thank you for educating me about the importance of breathing.

Lindsey Simms, Yvonne Kurant, Peter Howie and Alison Sherk who are not only co-workers but also good friends who generously gave me their time and feedback.

McArthur and Company for breathing life into the development and progression of this project. Kim, I cannot thank you enough for seeing the potential in this book and sharing my vision for a more natural, sustainable and ethical way of living. Ann, Devon and Kendra, thank you all for your thoroughness and warmth, which has taken so much of the anxiety out of being a first-time author.

My agent, Alisha Sevigny, for her passion and enthusiasm. Responding to emails even while on her honeymoon demonstrated more dedication than I could have ever wished for.

My partner Benjamin who has cooled my most heated and self-frustrated moments with his kindness and patience.

All of the Pure + Simple staff, made up of such talented and educated practitioners and coordinators, who have helped me learn so much about beauty as well as team building.

Beauty: Pure + Simple

A HOLISTIC GUIDE TO NATURAL BEAUTY

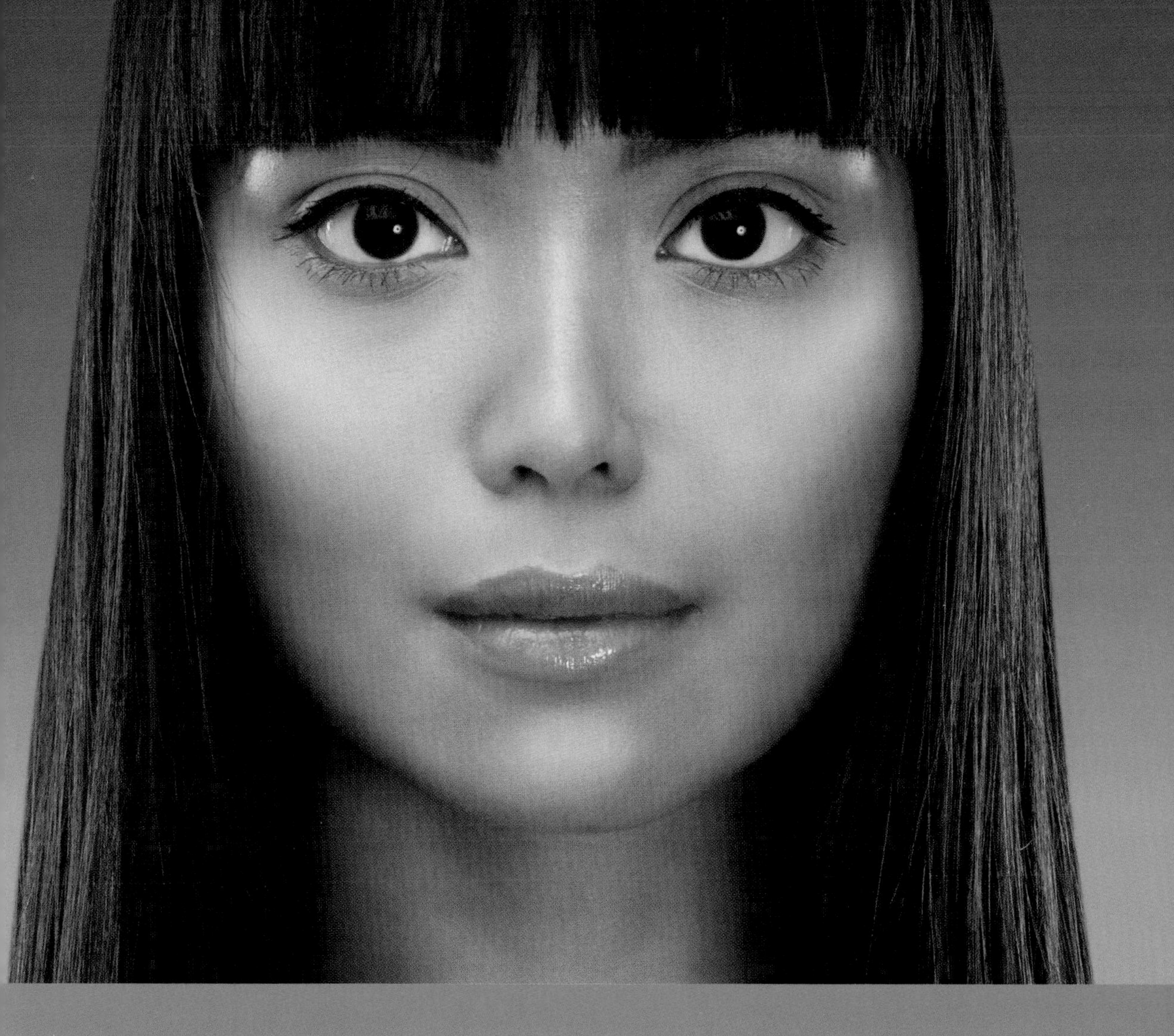

KRISTEN MA

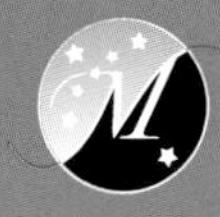

McArthur & Company
Toronto

First published by McArthur & Company in 2010

McArthur & Company
322 King Street West, Suite 402
Toronto, Ontario
M5V 1J2
www.mcarthur-co.com

Library and Archives Canada Cataloguing in Publication

Ma, Kristen
    Beauty pure + simple : a holistic guide to natural beauty / Kristen Ma.

Includes bibliographical references and index.
ISBN 978-1-55278-838-7

1. Skin–Care and hygiene. 2. Medicine, Ayurvedic. 3. Beauty, Personal.
4. Health. I. Title. II. Title: Beauty pure and simple.

RL87.M2 2010   646.7'26   C2009-907084-7

The publisher would like to acknowledge the financial support of the Government of Canada through the Book Publishing Industry Development Program (BPIDP) and the Canada Council for our publishing activities. The publisher further wishes to acknowledge the financial support of the Ontario Arts Council and the OMDC for our publishing program.

Cover design by Tania Craan
Typeset by Mary Bowness

Printed in Canada by Transcontinental Printing

10 9 8 7 6 5 4 3 2 1

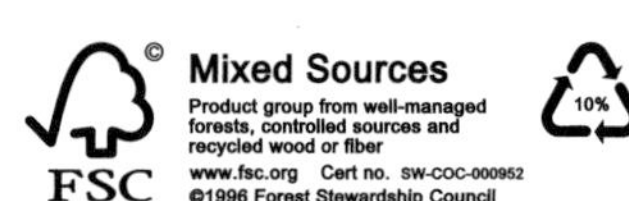

CONTENTS

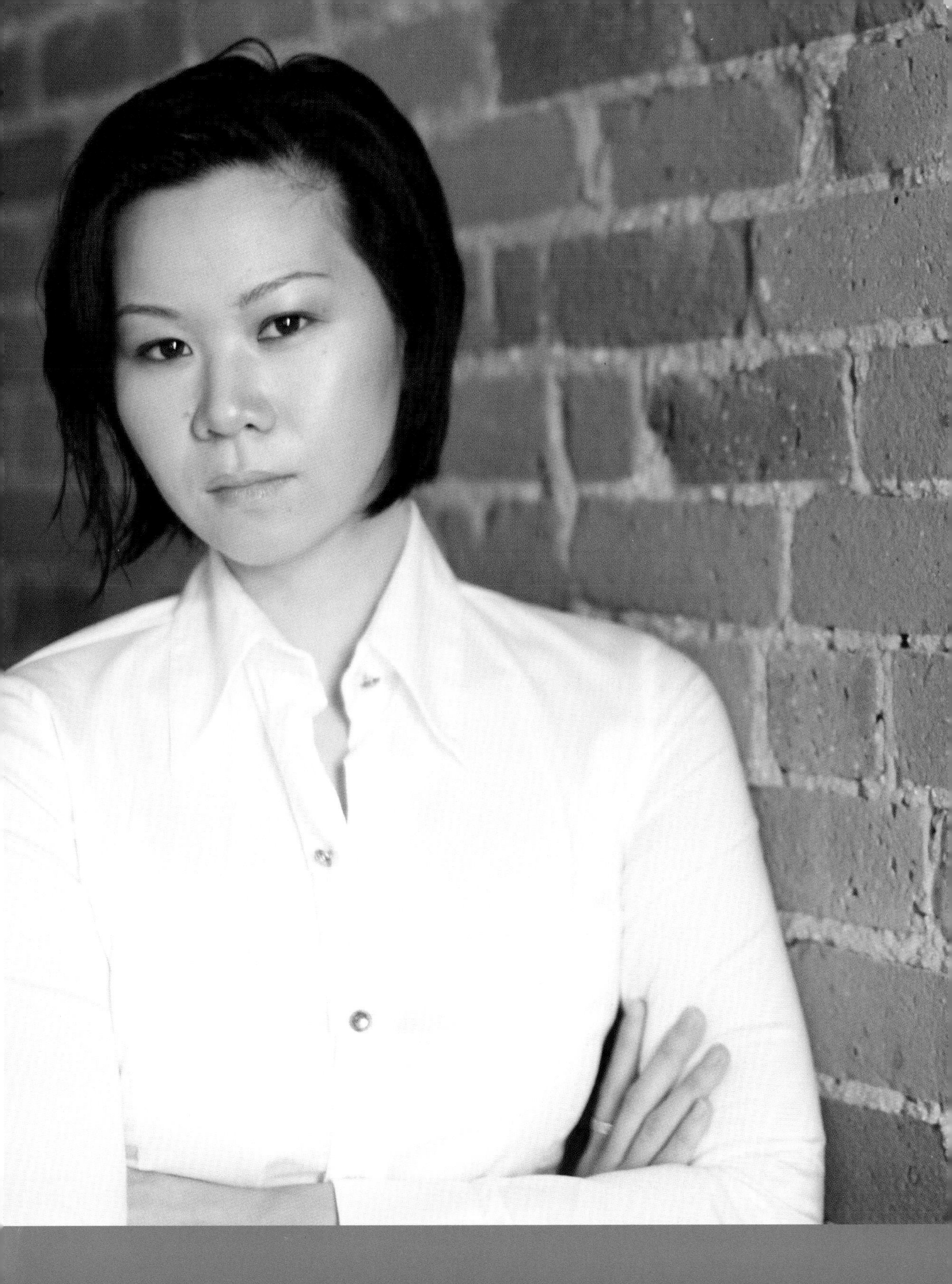

INTRODUCTION

The Pure + Simple Concept
A Different Definition of Beauty

Beauty in the Modern Age: High Expectations

In this competitive modern age, we have high expectations. Not only do we demand top performance from our products, services and technologies, but we also demand this of ourselves. Most of us strive to be the best in our jobs, our relationships, as parents, as children, as partners, as hosts, as managers and as members of our communities. Naturally, our attitude toward how we look is just as uncompromising.

In placing these expectations on ourselves, we sometimes forget what beauty really is and how best to embody it.

In my ten years as an esthetician, I have seen two very different sides to the promotion of beauty. One emphasizes traits like glowing skin, shiny hair, bright eyes and strong bodies, which can only come from balanced good health inside and out, making us innately magnetic and disarming.

Unfortunately, the other side of beauty is promoted as something very different from health – as a straighter, smaller nose, bigger breasts, poutier lips and taut skin. It is a rigid definition which supports the idea that beauty can be attained synthetically, through fake nails, fake hair, fake tans and fake eyelashes. This preference for external perfection over well-being also leads to the usage of dangerous procedures which damage, rather than enhance our health, and especially our skin.

It was this dichotomy that led my mother, Jean Eng, and I to start Pure + Simple Inc., a chain of holistic spas along with our own line of natural skincare and mineral makeup. Pure + Simple's mandate was to offer alternatives to conventional products and treatments for a more healthy attainment of beauty. These alternatives were not only in the form of chemical-free skincare, but also as skin consultations which took inside-outside beauty into account. After a few years of operation, I decided to further strengthen my understanding of the connection between health and beauty by becoming an Ayurvedic practitioner.

Ayurveda is a 5,000-year-old East Indian Science of Health and Medicine which teaches that healing (and, therefore, beauty) stems from a balanced lifestyle supported by knowledge. It is based on the concept that our bodies are composed of three different energies: Pitta, heat energy; Kapha, water and earth energy; and Vata, air and space energy. It is not the breakdown of our physical systems that causes sickness, but an excess or deficiency of a specific energy that imbalances and compromises our total selves.

One principle that runs consistently through all Eastern medicine is the idea that we must participate in our own well-being instead of hoping for someone, or something else, to save us. Whether it is a drug, a surgical procedure or the expertise of a practitioner, many of us expect external intervention to heal us, placing little thought on how we, ourselves, can contribute. This viewpoint also applies to beauty. Ayurveda promotes a more proactive approach, placing the emphasis on prevention instead of on short-term solutions that merely suppress our symptoms. Many of us suffer from acne, rosacea and eczema, hyper-pigmentation and premature aging, which may seem like ugly nuisances, but they are, in fact, early-warning signs of potentially more serious problems. If we treat these imperfections as a spur to change, we will not only gain beautiful skin but better health and greater vitality.

In particular, Ayurveda relies on daily care to deal with symptoms we deem unsightly by addressing their underlying cause. By contrast, current Western culture often encourages us to neglect this responsibility with its inherent respect for ourselves, opting instead for acute, drastic treatments in pursuit of false ideals. These unloving procedures, intended to reduce fine lines, to tone or even reconstruct features, are often counterproductive since they tax our bodies, our minds, our emotions and our immune systems. To be truly beautiful, it is important that we see this quality as something we want to develop, not as something external we want to obtain by artificial means.

The repercussions from treating our skin with severity can be long-lasting. The skin is an intimate and delicate organ with its own internal system. While many people think of it as just what they see, it is composed of three layers of tissue, each with its own sub-layers. Together they encapsulate a network of capillaries and sweat glands bound by tightly woven fibers of collagen and elastin. Understanding how complex and fragile our skin is can help us to make more informed choices.

I have an expanding clientele made up of people who did not initially have this understanding and who made rash decisions with the help of medical professionals. Many have induced adult skin conditions which are a direct result of having treated teenage acne with harsh peels, medications and drying agents prescribed by dermatologists or other doctors. These band-aid solutions typically produced short-term results accompanied by long-term damage such as skin sensitivity, dehydration and mental stress.

I, too, was someone who did this to my skin. I suffered from acne for more than ten years, for which I desperately searched for a solution, spending endless amounts of money and energy on my stubbornly blemished face. I religiously tried dry ice, glycolic peels and salicylic acid, making my skin red and creating scars (that I still have today). When this seemed insufficient, I took antibiotics, which not only made me feel ill, but which dried out my skin and internal organs.

I often compare this struggle to a war. I was fighting acne by peeling, drying and extracting as if it were an outside enemy and not a part of me. It was only when I started to treat myself with natural skincare that I began to see a difference. Though I had not really believed such a simple solution would be effective, I had exhausted most other avenues and was willing to try anything.

At first, I achieved only the lessening of my skin's redness, but in time my whole face began to look moister and healthier. While I still had blemishes, they looked calmer and less aggravated. This motivated me to shift from using "oil-free" and "purifying" products to natural, nourishing ones that targeted sensitivity and dehydration. That was when my skin became more balanced and I began to break out less. At that point, I became inspired to take initiative with my internal health by doing a series of detoxes and diet shifts, later offering the results of my findings to others.

All this is why I love natural beauty care. Not only did I clear up my skin and increase my self-confidence, but I learned how to treat myself gently and to love myself. Now, along with more attractive skin, I have a new perspective on myself and on how both the mind and the internal body affect the skin. I only wish I had received better guidance and learned these things earlier!

Knowledge is beauty

The reason many of us make mistakes when choosing our health and beautycare is that we are driven by fear: fear we are not attractive, fear people do not like us, fear we cannot achieve our goals. According to Ayurveda, fear not only affects the function of our kidneys but it also prevents us from moving forward positively. Today, very critical events are occurring in our world and in the environment requiring us to act. We need to feel empowered and that can only come from knowledge because knowledge *is* power.

When I was growing up, my mother always said: "Kristen, people can steal your things, whether it is a car, a watch or even your husband, but they can't take away what's in your mind – knowledge and wisdom are your most important investment."

But, acquiring knowledge about how to treat the skin can be very difficult. There is so much information to wade through on cosmetics and skincare products, while a large amount of it is conflicting. Despite all this clutter from the promotion of various lotions and potions – across the counter, at the spa, in the drugstore and on the Internet – we often are not told what we really need to know, such as which products contain caustic or even toxic ingredients.

Petroleum (a petrochemical often used as a product base) does not fully absorb into the skin, leaving it undernourished and clogging pores. This causes acne, blackheads and allergic reactions. Sodium laurel sulfate (SLS, used in detergents) is a stripping agent that dehydrates the skin and imbalances its acid mantle, aggravating sensitivity and preventing it from healing properly. Both products can also cause internal damage when absorbed into our bodies through our skin.

While there are other ingredients to avoid, these two are the most common. Conversely, pure ingredients, which feed and heal our skin, are increasingly accessible as the market itself becomes more aware.

When my mother and I first launched Pure + Simple a decade ago, natural skincare was not in vogue. We had to do a lot of educating, and many of our clients were initially skeptical; however, as more of them saw tangible results in their own complexions and told others, the demand for natural beauty flourished.

Avoiding harmful ingredients and choosing healthy ones is only part of the solution. At Pure + Simple we believe in coupling this with a balanced lifestyle. Through this book, I want to help others care for themselves in a way that allows them to feel beautiful and vibrant, with glowing skin as a result. I hope that by encouraging a healthy approach to self-image we can reexamine our outlooks, emphasizing the positive, so that we can make effective changes in our lives and in the world.

I base these hopes on the fact that many clients have already told me that Pure + Simple has changed their lives. I am honoured (and encouraged) to hear this because it is my intention to go beyond merely promoting wonderful creams and teach the proven knowledge and intuition of Ayurveda. By listening to our bodies and choosing appropriate actions, we can increasingly look and feel our best. Nothing is more attractive than a self-empowered person who is healthy in mind, body and spirit.

Beauty in Moderation

We at Pure + Simple are modernists with a practical, realistic outlook. While we promote natural skincare, we keep in mind differing goals and challenges. When our clients resort to chemical medications or invasive surgeries, we use our knowledge to help them to compensate for side-effects and unforeseen consequences in the best way possible because we believe that being judgmental or uncompromising is also unhealthy.

Everything on this earth can be a poison or a cure, depending on what and who we are treating. For example, in contrast to popular Western belief, Eastern medicine teaches that some of us need the stimulation of smoking (Kaphas) and the heaviness of starchy carbohydrates (Vatas), while others cannot take the over-stimulation of regular cardio exercise (Pittas and Vatas). Balance is everything.

This philosophy is extended to how we view beauty treatments. While many purists insist that basic facials and good creams are enough to heal any ailment, we believe that some aggressive, yet non-invasive procedures, if done conscientiously, can be extremely beneficial for the skin. This is especially true for those looking for anti-aging results.

Modern procedures like IPL (intense pulsed light), LED (light emitting diode) and Sea-salt Microdermabrasion can eliminate pigmented spots and the visible effects of broken capillaries, as well as minimizing fine lines. Skincare and massage alone cannot yield the results of these more stimulating treatments.

But proper selection and customization of these services are what will be truly effective. Sifting through the array of different skincare treatments and products can be made much simpler by choosing those that are specific to our Ayurvedic constitution. It is this pairing of new technology with ancient methodology that shapes Pure + Simple's approach.

Beauty in Simplicity

Our bodies are worlds within worlds! Each is a holistic system containing seven interconnected subordinate systems: circulatory, nervous, endocrine, muscular, lymphatic, digestive and skeletal. It is this complexity that makes knowing what is healthy so difficult. Add the fact that each of us is a unique individual so that no one solution can be good for everyone. That is why I always tell my clients they are the experts when it comes to themselves. They have been with themselves 24 hours a day for their whole lives. My job is to listen while providing additional knowledge and support.

I found my own search for health and beauty very exasperating because different experts touted different studies and opinions about what was good and bad. I came to the point where I felt I could not eat anything or follow any advice without feeling I was second-guessing myself. Simply sustaining myself had become overwhelming.

By writing this book, I hope that my own hard-won research will be used as a tool and as a resource to help others find solace in holistic and natural ways. Along with normal skincare and maintenance, I will tell you about the three basic principles I found that I could apply to everything, from the search for beauty to emotional exploration - moving, purging and nourishing. For those of us who are reformed skin-abusers, I will also discuss how to repair damage that has already occurred, along with the best ways to internally and externally treat ailments like acne, sensitivity, rosacea, eczema, hyper-pigmentation and signs of aging (tissue degeneration). This book is also a compilation of knowledge that we at Pure + Simple wish to pass on to those of you who, at present, are just browsing, in hopes that you, too, will be inspired to embrace the Ayurvedic process of beautification.

Many of my clients came to Pure + Simple much like beauty refugees searching for a positive and healthy way to look and feel good. We offer a more nurturing option: skincare which is gentle and nourishing, using pure ingredients, along with the knowledge that fosters positive choices. This is the approach we have employed for the past decade, and is what we are known for.

Kristen Ma

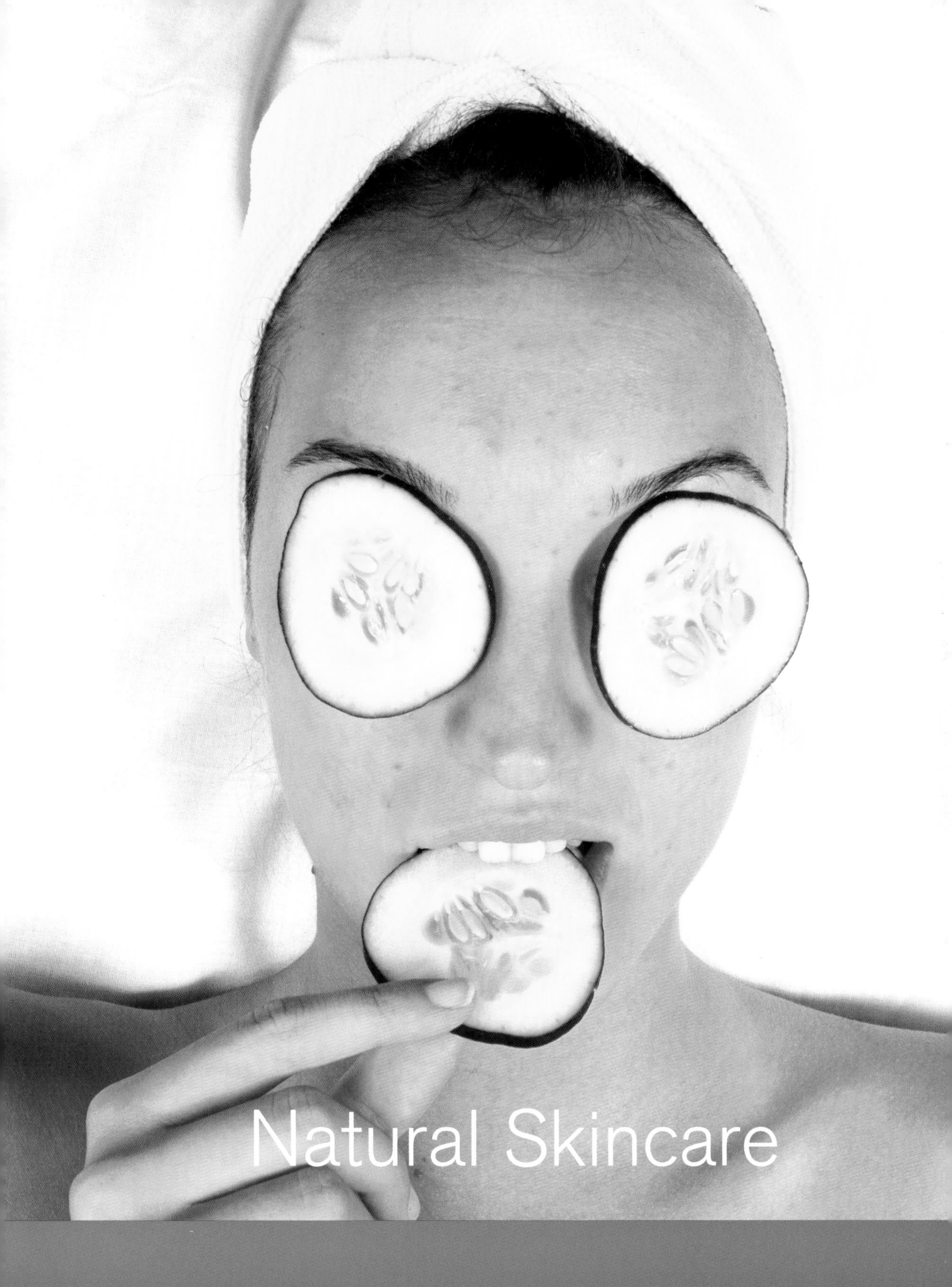

Natural Skincare

CHAPTER 1

What is Natural Skincare?

The definition for natural skincare products has become clouded. Cosmetic marketers label products as "natural" when they contain as little as two per cent natural ingredients. Unfortunately, consumers assume this labeling ensures complete natural content.

Reasons to go Natural

There has been a lot of hype about natural and organic beauty products, but what exactly are the benefits? Why go natural? Why spend the extra money and effort to sort through the cluttered world of cosmetics? How do you tell which product lines are actually natural, and which are just capitalizing on the trend?

During my years in the beauty industry, I have seen the progress my clients have made with natural skincare compared to those who use chemical brands. Some people consider natural ingredients less potent in their effects, but my own battle with acne gave me firsthand experience that chemically-based skincare brands do not produce a sustainable long-term solution.

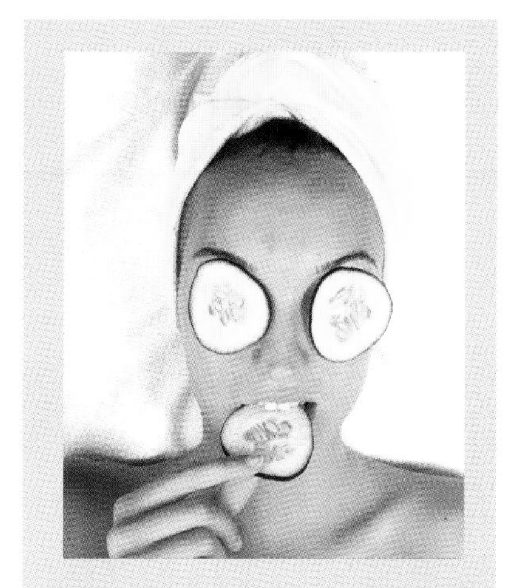

A more accurate definition of a natural skincare product would be one that:

1. Contains at least 95 per cent fully natural ingredients.
2. Possesses no ingredients with a potential or suspected health risk.
3. Uses no processes that significantly or adversely alter the purity or the effect of the natural ingredients.

10 Reasons to Go Natural

1. **Support ethical companies**
   Support smaller skincare companies which utilize ethical practices, higher quality ingredients and honest marketing.
2. **Endorse humane treatment of animals**
   Endorse cruelty-free skincare and makeup.
3. **Support a natural environment**
   Support an environment free of toxic chemicals and pesticides. Stop the pollution and depletion of the earth's soil and the use of genetic engineering.
4. **Soothe Sensitivity**
   Aid sensitivity through natural products, as chemical ingredients cause skin irritation and allergic reactions.
5. **Stop clogging**
   Stop clogging pores by using petroleum-free skincare. Petroleum-based products cannot fully penetrate the skin and sit on the skin's surface causing acne, dehydration and blackheads
6. **Prevent Aging**
   Prevent aging by using vegetable-based skincare which fully penetrates the skin. This eliminates dehydration and fine lines as these product can truly hydrate and nourish.
7. **Protect your health**
   Protect your health with skincare which is free of toxic chemicals. Prevent the absorption of harmful and carcinogenic ingredients into the skin, body tissues and bloodstream.
8. **Go holistic**
   Go with a holistic view of the body, mind and spirit. Embrace a more natural definition of beauty, including that of your mental and emotional state. Realize the skin is a reflection of the internal.
9. **Feed your skin**
   Feed your skin for a healthy glow. Natural products boost the skin's own defense system, aiding skin ailments such as eczema, rosacea and dermatitis.
10. **Detoxify**
    Detoxify your skin and body. Clogged pores inhibit detoxification through perspiration. The body is also enabled to purge toxins, as it is no longer taxed by harmful chemicals, dyes and perfumes.

Natural Skincare for More Beautiful, Healthier Skin

Natural products use pure vegetable and plant oils, waters and waxes as their base, whereas conventional product lines use petroleum (mineral oil, petrolatum, propylene glycol, etc.). Our skin loves (and deeply absorbs) natural ingredients. It does not like petrochemicals and acts as a gatekeeper to limit their harmful effects.

Prevent Pore Congestion

Since petroleum molecules are too large to fully penetrate the skin, products containing them clog the pores and suffocate the skin. This causes outbreaks of acne and blackheads, preventing the skin from absorbing moisture – both from our skincare and the humidity in the air.

This realization often provides an "eureka" moment for my clients, who have tried countless moisturizers only to discover that they sit on their skin's surface without penetrating. One client, a PhD biochemistry student, had explored everything from the science of hormones to high-tech skincare. She was at her wits end, having spent so much money and tried so many approaches, none of which had stopped her acne breakouts. She was using medicated creams from her dermatologist containing benzoyl peroxide and salicylic acid, which dried her skin, making it flaky and irritated. She did not have oily skin, but dry, sensitive skin which was being further dehydrated by the acne-targeting products that unbalanced her oil production and clogged her pores.

I explained the absorption of natural ingredients to her, then prescribed a gentle, restorative regime consisting of multiple moisturizers and Pure + Simple's Sensitive Skin Face Oil. When she returned, she brought me flowers to thank me for changing her understanding of beautycare. Today, her skin is completely clear and she uses an oil-rich moisturizing cream mask daily to repair her skin's sensitivity.

Stop Stripping the Skin

Chemical detergents in conventional skincare strip and deplete the skin's acid mantle, leaving it damaged, vulnerable and prone to reactions like over-sensitivity and oil imbalance. While many of us understand that treating our skin harshly will aggravate sensitive skin and dry out dehydrated skin, we do not understand that stripping the skin is actually a contributor to break outs and black heads as well.

Nourish the Skin

Some companies combine natural ingredients with chemically-based thickeners. This enables the product to consist mostly of water with very little nourishing properties. Truly natural skincare products use only ingredients which fully penetrate to feed the skin, along with cleansing agents which gently remove dirt. This nourishes, protects and heals existing damage. The skin is an organ which needs to be pampered and handled with care.

Natural Skincare for a Healthier Body

As we all know, beauty is more than skin deep. True beauty is the reflection of a healthy mind and body. Nothing is more attractive than someone who radiates vitality.

We Absorb Everything that is on Our Skin

All products applied onto our skin absorb into our blood stream and internal organs. Therefore, products containing toxic chemicals will affect our overall health. Our sunscreens, our makeup and our skincare products often contain carcinogenic ingredients which eventually damage us in ways we would never have suspected. For example, certain sunscreen agents imbalance our hormonal system, and some chemical ingredients tax our kidneys and liver, yet we rub these into our bodies on a habitual basis.

Containers and Packaging of Beauty Products can affect our Health

Many of us neglect to assess the packaging our products are contained in. But since the residues and leakage from various plastics can be toxic, using glass and food-grade plastics is important. Remember, all of the principles we apply to skincare ingredients also apply to materials which interact with them. This is why many companies have become much more holistic in their product development and design. Organic German line, Martina Gebhardt, uses only ceramic packaging because it is nontoxic, maintains the purity of their products, and is a more sustainable material.

Natural Skincare Encourages Self-Awareness

Interest in natural skincare and holistic beauty leads to increased self-awareness, putting us more in tune with the changes in our bodies. I continually encourage my clients to notice what happens to their breathing and heart rate when they experience stress. I teach them to change their skincare when the weather changes to respond to the environment around them. I also offer dietary advice.

When clients learn to use diet, skincare and stress-relief to balance their bodies, they become more aware of monitoring themselves. They also become more aware of the relationship between the mind, the body, their emotions and their surroundings.

Natural Skincare Encourages Social Responsibility

I was never very interested in the beauty industry until I understood its link to wellness. While I found grooming the perfect brow and shaping graceful nails to be fun, these esthetics on their own were not something to which I wanted to devote my life. The broader picture – teaching people how to love themselves and to be more conscious of their bodies – was what I really wanted to endorse.

Personal beauty is only fulfilling when we also encourage more beauty in our environment. To be gorgeous inside and out means being conscious of how we consume, and what ideas we promote. Our values on beauty greatly reflect who we are and what beliefs we support.

Caring for ourselves this way is empowering. Using skincare products which are healthy for our bodies as well as our skin results in a holistic view of ourselves and of beauty.

We are a System

Progress does not come through preaching alone. How we behave as individuals makes a larger impact than simply advertising our principles.

Working for ethical companies and buying socially responsible products makes a powerful statement about how we view the environment. Biodegradable products have a synergy with the Earth. What we wash from our bodies or eliminate, we put into the world's ecosystem. Antidepressants, hormones and plasticides have been found in drinking water, passed there through our urine. This was noted in the 1980s when fish species in the St. Lawrence River began to display gender changes. These fish were found to have both eggs and testes. A study in which these fish were fed to lab rats showed that over time, the rats too, also displayed hormone imbalances. We must realize what an impact our consumption has on our ecosystem as well as the circularity of our world.

Sustainable Packaging

As mentioned before, packaging should play an integral role to our shopping decisions. Not only can it affect the safety of a product, but also adds to the waste accumulated in our environment. We must limit the use of packaging and also use renewable materials.

We at Pure + Simple do not use boxes in our packaging because they are wasteful and excessive. We use glass containers for purity and sustainability. We also have a bottle-return service (as more and more companies are doing), cutting costs as well as waste.

When we as humans produce goods on a large scale, we deplete the Earth's resources, greatly affecting our planet's future. At a Green Enterprise event I attended on behalf of Pure + Simple, environmentalist Paul Hawkin said: "Any time someone steals something from our future, it is injustice.... We steal from the future and sell it in the present and call it GDP." This was very inspiring to me. We must realize that industry and pollution can no longer be intertwined. One of the most effective ways to change and communicate this is through making more conscious buying decisions.

Respecting the Environmental Landscape

Respecting the planet does not have to mean letting go of our vanity, but does require indulging ourselves with a sense of responsibility. Just Pure, Jurlique, Martina Gebhardt and Dr. Hauschka Skincare farm their ingredients respectfully by giving their land a cyclical rest so as not to deplete its fertility. They use biodynamic farming to replenish the soil and refrain from pesticides which would disturb its natural insect life. The traditional agricultural practices used to farm organics actually build carbon back into the soil.

Support Ethics

Promoting positive ideas and business practices are the first stage of changing counterproductive social habits. Doing this includes supporting companies that care about their customers' well-being, and encouraging even more of them to include this in their corporate missions. Buying natural skincare is not only better for our skin and bodies, but also endorses businesses which put the health of their customers first.

Promoting a Healthy and Practical View of Beauty

A healthy and practical perception of beauty is important for our society. We must stop wishing we were someone else, pining for the perfect cheek bones, lips, hips and breasts and believing that artificial characteristics are ideal. Loving and accepting our humanness, instead of fixating on fragments of ourselves, is integral to developing a healthy outlook. Cosmetic companies that help their clients enhance their natural beauty foster these ideas and make the concept of beauty attainable for everyone.

As the basis for a forward-looking vision of inner and outer beauty, I would like to explain how our skin works, along with the tools for achieving that goal.

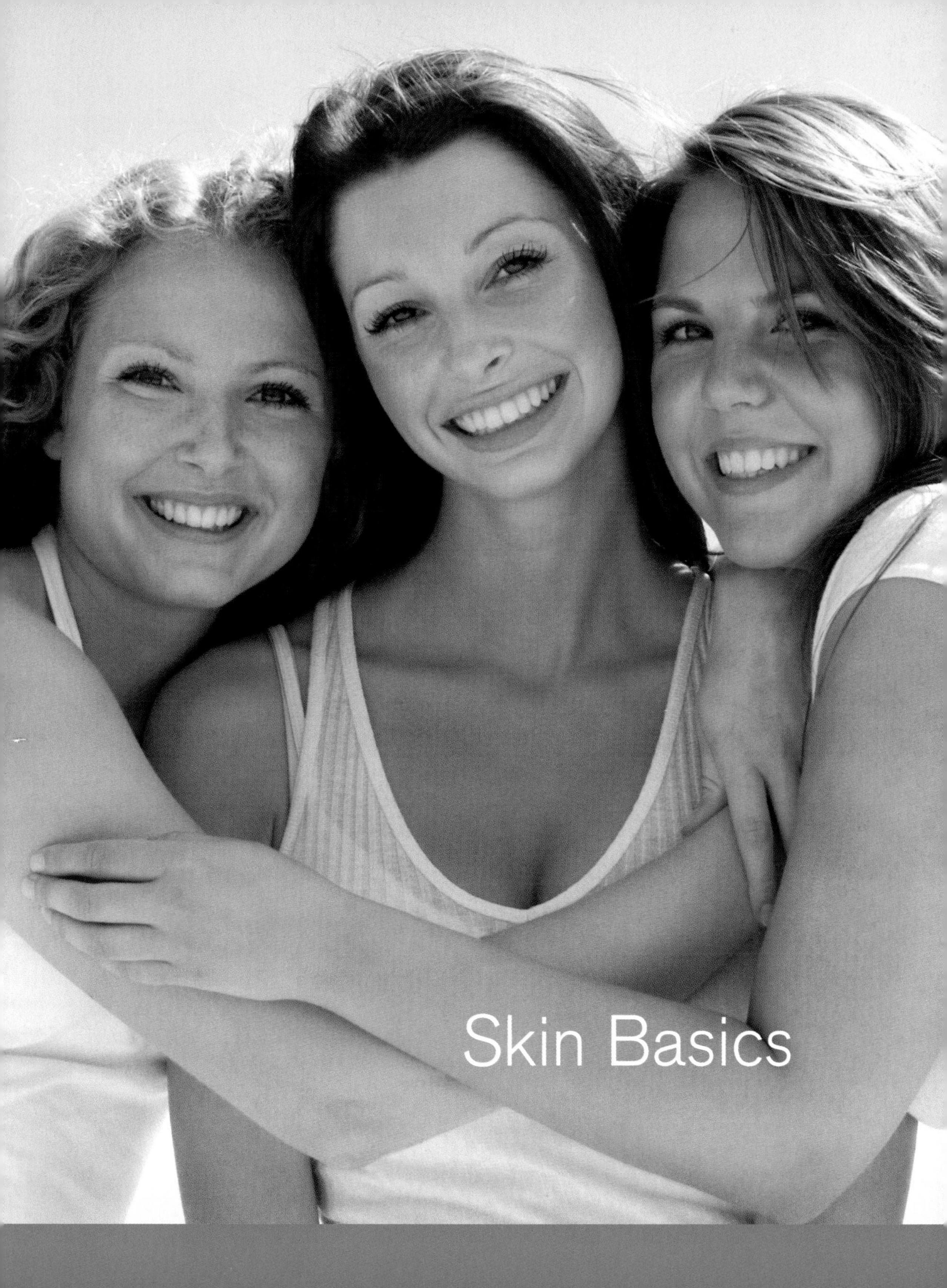

Skin Basics

CHAPTER 2

Understanding the Body's Largest Organ

Functions of the Skin

We usually judge our skin from an aesthetic viewpoint instead of appreciating it as our body's largest organ. Often we abuse it with harsh products and chemical peels, or by accidentally bumping, bruising, scraping and cutting it without any real awareness of the stress this puts on this valuable body shield. Fortunately, our skin has amazing self-repairing abilities.

Detoxification

The skin helps us detoxify by sweating and excreting sebum (oil), but many of us prevent this with pore-clogging products. Furthermore, most antiperspirants contain aluminum, which is toxic, and we thoughtlessly apply this to our underarms where there is a gathering of lymph nodes important for detoxification and the fighting of disease. While this is socially encouraged, it inhibits a process which is integral to our overall health. By contrast, dry-brushing and body exfoliation aid detoxification through our pores while reducing cellulite.

Since the capillaries in our skin also transport away debris such as bacteria, pollution, dead cells and absorbed skincare ingredients, keeping the walls of our blood vessels supple is important to detoxification.

The Skin Breathes

A small percentage of our total oxygen intake is absorbed through our pores. When they are clogged, the skin looks devitalized and the decrease in oxygen contributes to signs of aging. This has led to the popularization of antioxidants. Using natural skincare and having regular facials to extract congestion is necessary both for the skin and our overall health.

Regulating Body Temperature

The skin regulates our body heat. When we are too hot, the skin opens pores to release heat. This is called vasodilation. When we are cold, the body closes up pores, trapping in heat. This is called vasoconstriction. Vasoconstriction is the cause of what is referred to as *goosebumps*. When the pores tighten they form a bump and cause the hair to stand on end.

Tactile Sensing and Touch

The skin contains sensory nerves which govern touch. It is through our skin that we feel textures and consistencies. A calming massage not only soothes the skin but also harmonizes the mind.

Reflecting Emotional States

When we are embarrassed, we blush. When we are shocked, we turn pale. Since the skin is a mirror of our emotions, it is not surprising that its ailments often have emotional triggers. From my own experience, I know that stress is the main cause of my eczema outbreaks. Many of my rosacea clients also say stress causes their flare-ups. One of my clients, who is a student, gets a rash on her elbows during exams like clockwork. Forehead lines, dehydration and acne are also related to anxiety and other forms of emotional distress. This will be discussed, in-depth, later in this book.

Protection

The skin is our body's armour. It protects our muscles, nerves and internal organs, and is the container for all our other systems. It also controls what passes in and out of our body, acting as its gatekeeper. Fortunately, it possesses a certain wisdom about toxic ingredients, preventing many of them from being fully absorbed. Without this supple, highly resilient shield we could not function.

Absorption

Since we absorb through our skin, we must choose carefully what we put on it. What is applied topically travels into the bloodstream through a network of capillaries connecting to larger vessels supplying the internal organs. The skin actually absorbs materials faster than the digestive system. What we eat must be processed before it fully affects our bodies, but anything applied to the skin has direct access to the bloodstream. A good example of this is provided by the nicotine patch which, when placed on the skin, allows nicotine into the body to wean us from our addictions. Some doctors also prescribe hormones through the application of creams. While we may think of beautycare as something topical, superficial and fun, its impact on our bodies as a holistic system is highly significant.

Examples of how quickly and deeply we absorb through our skin:

- To demonstrate the interconnectedness of the body, naturopathic schools conduct an exercise wherein they rub crushed garlic on the soles of participants' feet. Within twenty minutes, their breath will smell of garlic!

- When lavender essential oil is applied to the hands, traces of it will be found in the liver within half an hour.

- During a lecture at the Ayurvedic Academy at Bastyr University, Dr. Subhash Ranade spoke of an experiment conducted in an underprivileged village in India. Starvation had damaged the digestive systems of many children, making nutrition through eating difficult. As an alternative, these children were given a daily massage of milk infused with healing herbs, the absorption of which gradually restored the linings of their digestive tracts.

  Through the skin's absorption, the doctors made profound improvements in the children's weight and their digestive systems. I have never forgotten this beautiful story of how these children were nourished and nurtured back to health through massage.

The Skin's Structure

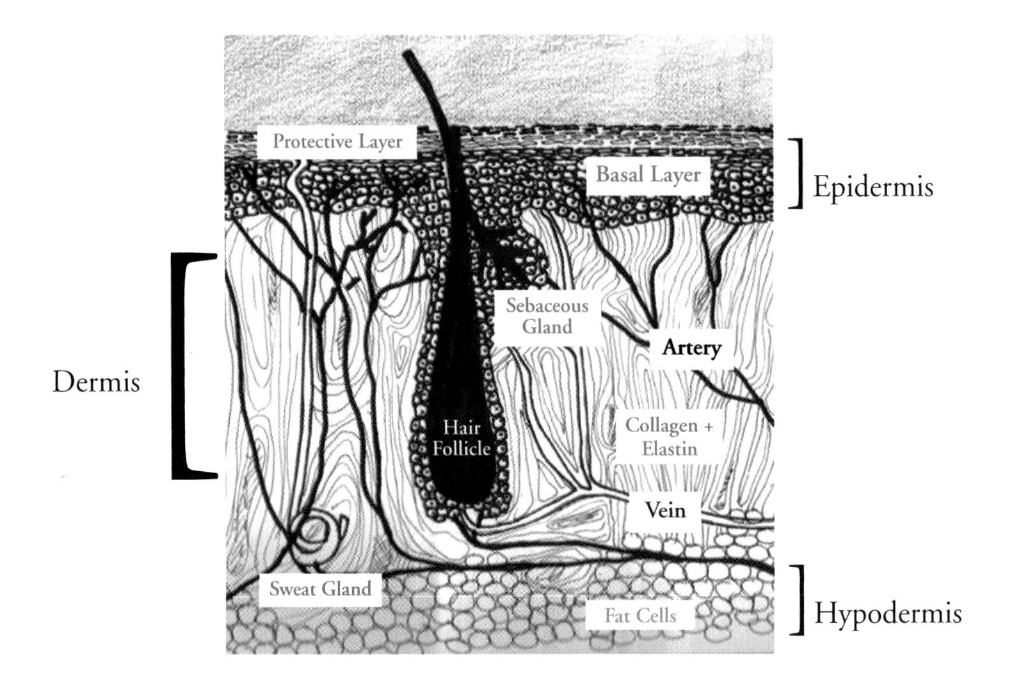

The Skin's Structure

To truly understand the skin and the part it plays in absorption and excretion, we must understand its makeup.

The Layers

Our skin is not just what we see but an entire factory, support system and shield for a variety of vitally functioning cells.

The skin is made up of three main layers: the epidermis, the dermis and the hypodermis (subcutaneous fatty tissue).

The Epidermis

The epidermis is the skin layer found closest to the surface. It is the outer shell which we see, and which acts as a barrier and a gateway. It comprises five layers of dead skin cells made up of keratin (protein). Keratinization is the process by which cells travel up through these layers to become the surface. It ends when these cells are sloughed off. The life cycle of a skin cell becomes slower and slower over the years, producing the effects we call aging.

The Dermis

The dermis is the main factory of the skin, containing our network of collagen and elastin fibers. Its connective tissue provides elasticity and nutrition to the epidermis. It is where our sweat and oil glands reside, excreting through the epidermis. It also contains the nerve endings which provide our sense of touch and temperature. Its health dictates the quality of the epidermis.

Hypodermis (subcutaneous fatty tissue)

This lowest layer of skin is the fatty cushion which insulates our bodies and protects our organs. Comprised primarily of fat and some connective tissue, it also possesses many skin-nourishing blood vessels and nerve endings.

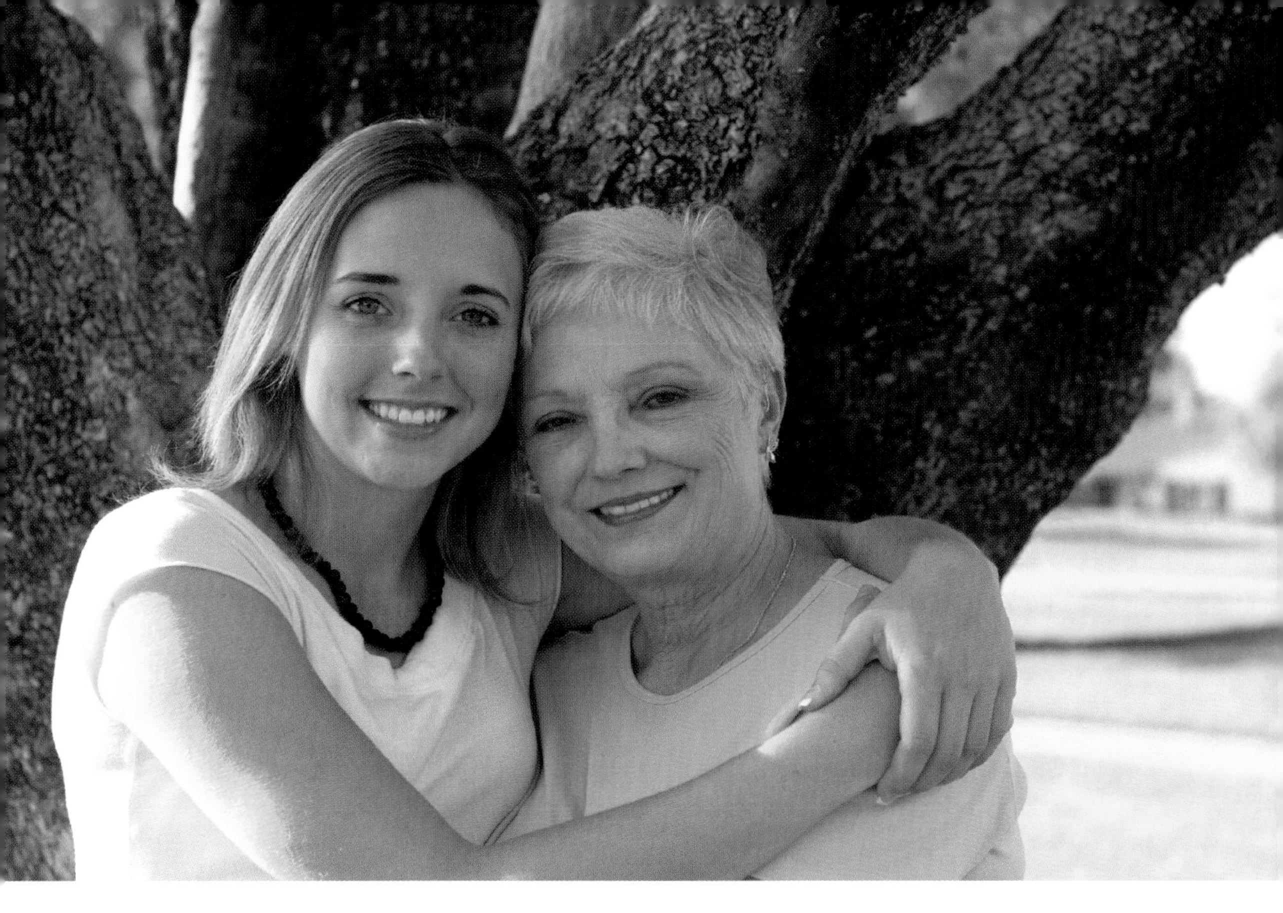

Aging and the Structure of the Skin

At the age of 25, the skin is at its peak of health. The dermis layer is thick, producing lots of plump, moist cells to be transferred to the epidermis. Cell turnover takes approximately *28* days.

As we age, our epidermis thickens, giving way to fine lines and wrinkles. Cell turnover slows **at age 45** to approximately *40* days. An accumulation of dead cells causes the skin to feel drier and to be less able to absorb moisture.

At age 75 and over, cell turnover drops to *90* days and metabolism and circulation slows down. An even thicker epidermal layer causes wrinkles to deepen, with the top layer forming a crust-like appearance.

These normal effects of aging have made skin peeling and abrasion popular. The erosion of the thickened epidermis causes the dermis to increase moisture and our skin to absorb it more deeply.

Skin Classification:
Skin, a Contingent Organ

To treat a problem, we need to classify and analyze it to find its root cause. Given that our bodies are so complex, and each of us so unique, we must design different treatments for each individual. This is the basis of Ayurveda. Each diagnosis is based on a person's original dosha (elemental constitution a.k.a. prakruti), along with the imbalance and differentiation that has developed from this origin. We will explore this topic in detail later. But first, let us examine the different ways to diagnose skin from an esthetician's viewpoint.

Conventional Classification: Skin Types

If you go to a department store cosmetic counter, they will base their suggestions on classic skin typing. Skin type refers to the genetic characteristic of our skin but does not take into account environmental or past regime factors. This classification alone is not effective in diagnosing the skin.

Dry Skin

Skin lacking in oil. Small pores, fine texture, possible leathery appearance in mature skin, no acne, possibly cysts.

Oily Skin

Excess oil on the skin's surface, enlarged pores, thick texture, deeper lines, acne-prone.

Combination Skin

Oily in some areas, dry in others, with corresponding textures.

Normal Skin

Balanced skin is referred to as normal. Ironically, while referred to as "normal," this skin type actually denotes a flawless complexion.

Skin Condition

While skin type describes what we inherited, skin conditions are acquired. This describes the state of the skin based on our environment and grooming history.

Dehydrated Skin

When skin is dehydrated, it is due to a lack of moisture. (Most of our skins are dehydrated.)

Sensitive Skin

While sensitive skin may be genetic, it is aggravated by the elements, diet, mindset and improper care. People with very allergic skin often have a lot of internal toxicity making their system delicate and their defenses weak.

Unbalanced Skin

Unbalanced skin is caused by drying, overactive adrenals or negligent skincare.

Problem Skin

Problem skin is not constituted by one or two pimples, but constant breakouts of acne or blemish clusters over the face and sometimes the neck. Causes vary from person to person. This will be discussed further in our Acne section.

Signs of dehydration:

- Crepey or crinkled texture
- Lack of colour
- Poor circulation
- Congested pores
- Skin tightness

Signs of sensitive skin:

- Redness
- Frequent blushing
- Broken capillaries
- Red allergy bumps
- A chaffed appearance

Signs of imbalanced skin:

- Oiliness and peeling
- Dryness or tightness and acne
- Oily skin with fine lines
- Congestion under the skin

Signs of problem skin:

- Whiteheads
- Blackheads
- Inflamed pimples
- Cysts

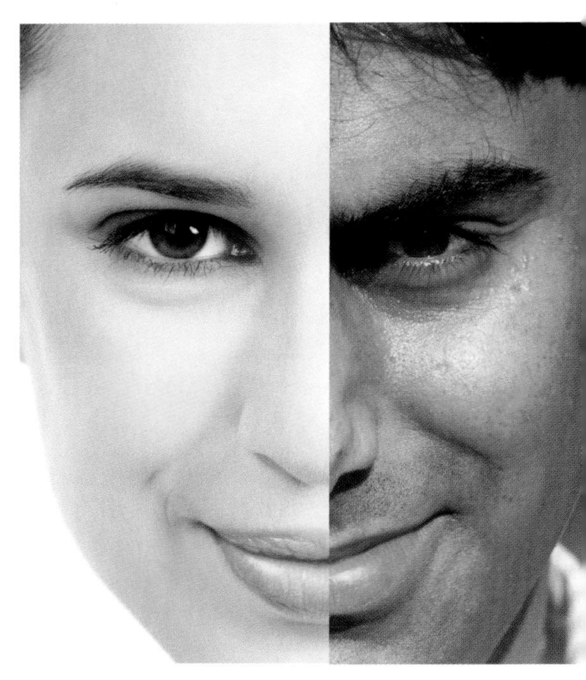

The Yin Yang of Skin: Female vs. Male Skin

Should skincare be sex specific?

While many grooming practices are gender neutral, some differences cannot be ignored.

Differences in the skin

Men have thicker skin. Most men also have tougher, rougher skin and even the most delicate male skin is much thicker and less sensitive than delicate female skin.

The male hormone testosterone increases collagen production, which is the main reason for the greater thickness. Estrogen decreases collagen synthesis but supports the presence of hyaluronic acid, which makes for a thinner, softer, texture.

While male skin owes much to physiology, men also have a skin-thickening, anti-aging practice ingrained in their grooming regimes since adolescence: *shaving.* As well as marking a rite of passage from boyhood to manhood, shaving is a first step in anti-aging treatments. This habitual exfoliation acts the same way as Microdermabrasion – it thickens the skin while it abrades it, causing regeneration. This is a major reason why men often have fewer fine lines and more vital skin.

Men also tend to have oilier skin. Because testosterone creates more active sebaceous glands, men are more likely to have acne and breakouts. Women with hormonal imbalances also share these attributes.

Female hormonal influences such as menstruation can cause breakouts, sensitivity and water retention. Many women experience acne breakouts before their period. According to Ayurveda, this is because both water and heat in the body are increased. Often they crave sweet, cooling foods, and have mood swings ranging from anger (heat-aggravated) to feelings of lethargy (water-aggravated). The skin's sensitivity is also heightened at this time.

Women are more likely to have rosacea, though its severe stages are usually only seen in men, due to their neglect of care. Water retention during menstruation also contributes to sensitivity because, if the lymph is full, the capillaries are pushed toward the skin's surface. This pressure can create broken capillaries, further increasing the skin's delicacy. For all these reasons, women who want beautiful skin must pay attention to their menstrual cycles.

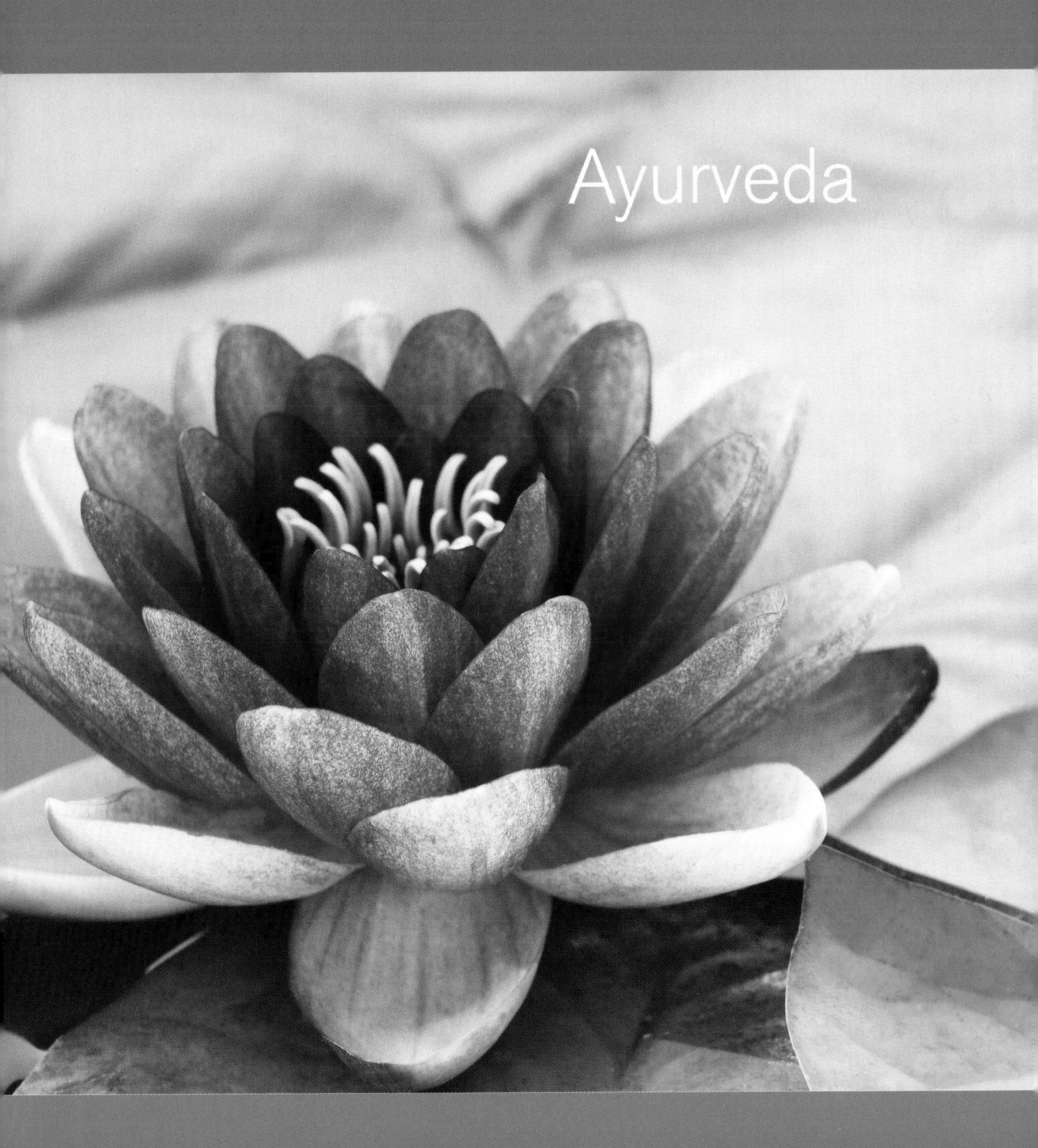

Ayurveda

CHAPTER 3

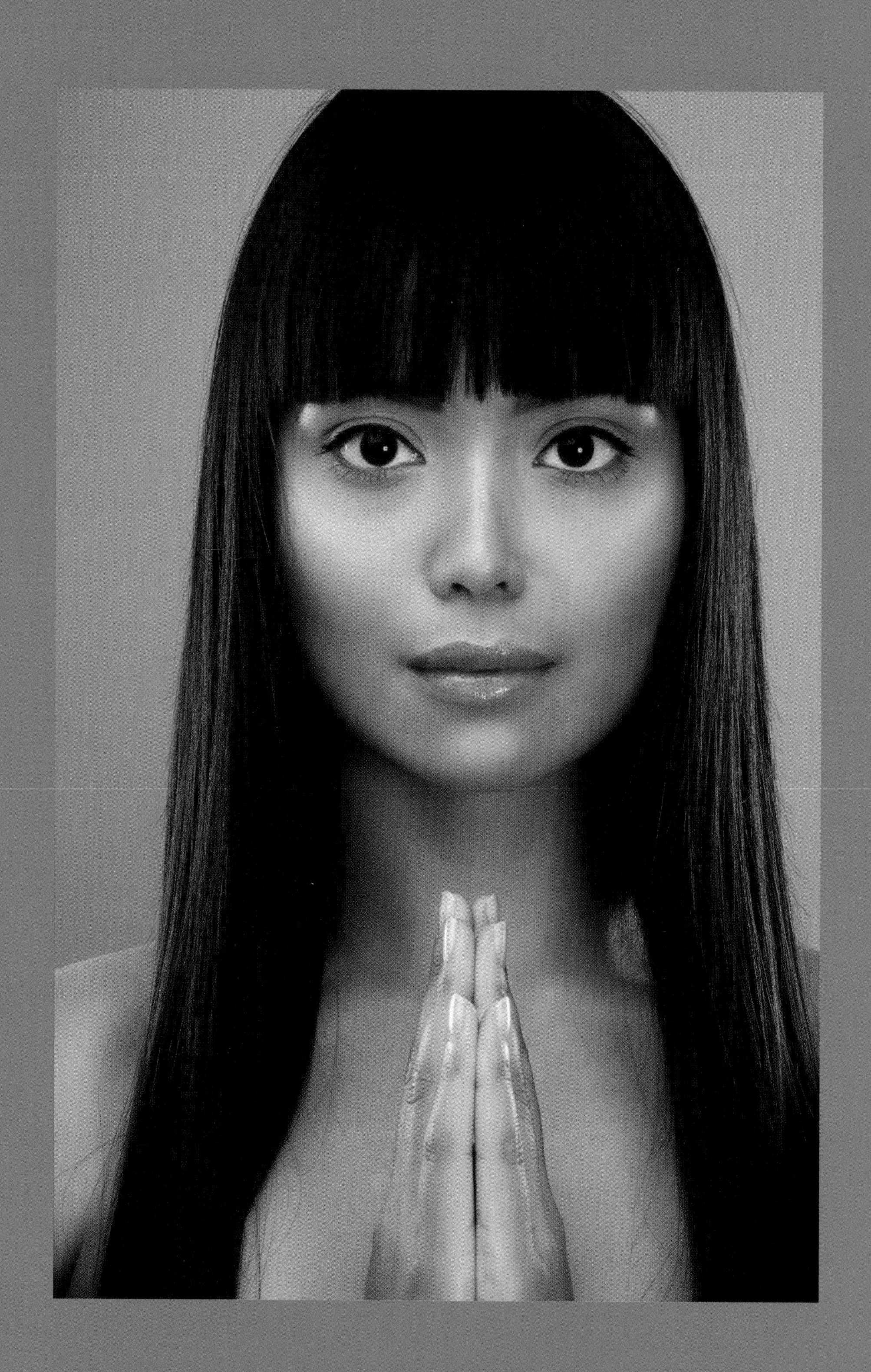

The Beauty of Eastern Medicine

I believe Ayurveda and Traditional Chinese Medicine (TCM) are very important in our pursuit of beautiful skin since these health systems focus on being preventative and holistic.

Most healing modalities, whether conventional or alternative, fail to offer a usable, consistent system which empowers the patient/client. Ayurveda's framework is so simple that every one of us can make daily choices for balancing our health in relation to our environment, constitution and own special needs. The spiritual dimension of both of these sciences also gives the user a beauty philosophy which profoundly supports maturing the mind and spirit.

Because I am an Ayurvedic practitioner, this book is heavily influenced by Ayurvedic philosophy, but it also contains TCM information. This explanation of health and beauty further demonstrates the mind, body and spirit connection.

Ayurveda

Ayurveda, literally translated, means *the science or study of life*. Its conception dates back 5,000 years to the Himalayans in Northern India.

Ayurveda guides us to live in harmony and beauty, according to our individual constitutions and our environment. It illustrates how each of us is a unique person with unique needs, perspective, personality, rate of digestion, speed of metabolism and so on. Therefore, it is logical that each of us must customize our treatments, diets and habits to maintain health, to feel beautiful and to live with vitality.

Since Ayurveda emphasizes prevention, we learn to become self-aware through listening to ourselves, our intuition and our bodies. Treating small imbalances can prevent an accumulation leading to disease, but this requires us to be responsible and proactive in our wellness, as well as taking an active role in our healing.

In India, Ayurvedic doctors are traditionally paid an annual block fee to treat their patients rather than on a case by case basis (and sometimes they are simply paid with whatever offering a patient has available to them). Since treating patients who are more ill requires more time and energy, this system encourages a proactive and preventative approach. Not only are they healers but they are also teachers who educate their patients on maintaining health and preventing disease. While Western surgeons are highly compensated for treating severe situations, Ayurvedic doctors are rewarded more for avoiding invasive procedures.

Ayurveda also has an entire branch of post-treatment rejuvenation (rasayana) utilizing therapies and medicines which restore the body. These practices are excellent for anti-aging as well.

Of course, I can provide only a snapshot of Ayurveda in this book, as it is a vast ideology with many factions; however, its basic principles will help readers develop a deeper understanding of health, balance and beauty.

How is Ayurvedic Healing Different than Western Medicine?

Western medicine (allopathic) often focuses on alleviating symptoms, treating pain, inflammation, tumors or depression with painkillers, anti-inflammatory drugs, antidepressants and surgeries. This approach ignores the source of the dysfunction. Ayurveda, in contrast, always searches for the root cause, and treats ailments from this perspective.

A parallel holds true for the achievement of beauty. Western treatments try to minimize the wrinkle, dry out the pimple and cover the redness without seeking out the imbalances creating them in lifestyle and behavior.

To understand ourselves as individuals, we must start by determining our constitutions – what Ayurveda calls *doshas*. These are the elements that we all possess: earth/water, fire and air. Though each of us have all three doshas within ourselves, it is the degree of each which makes us unique. Usually we will have one dominant dosha with the other two exerting a lesser influence; however, some of us have two main doshas, while rare individuals are tridoshic, meaning they have equal amounts of all three.

Once we know who we are, we can see and feel when our bodies are out of balance, diverting us from our natural states.

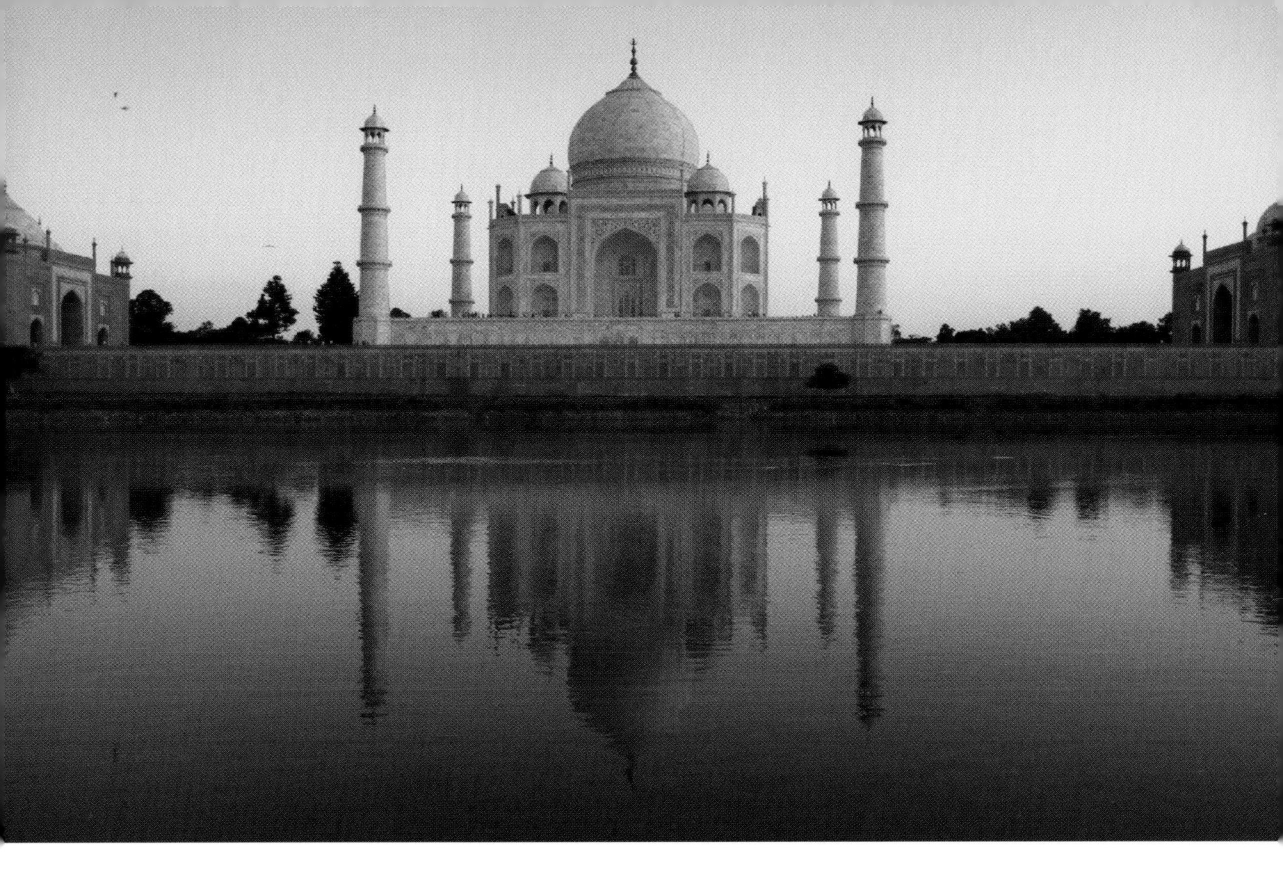

Ayurveda and Beauty

While I was in India, I was astonished by how much beauty was integrated into the culture. Even in poor or polluted communities, people still found ways of surrounding themselves with lovely things. They decorated their cars and trucks with bright, fresh-flower garlands bought from vendors, bringing colour to beaten-up streets. I loved how they used real flowers, with their lovely aromas, despite their fragility. And, of course, they were biodegradable.

Ayurveda is an incredibly romantic ideology. It encompasses love, sex and beauty as part of a healthy lifestyle. Caring for the skin and body is a daily Ayurvedic ritual, beginning with a morning self-massage, followed by cleansing and exfoliation with Ayurvedic herbs.

The key to understanding our health, hence our beauty, is in perceiving that everything about our minds, bodies and our environment is always changing. This means that our rituals and products must also change to accommodate this state of perpetual flux. What is good for one season is not good for another and the skincare and diet we adopted five years ago no longer suits the shifting landscape inside ourselves. Finding balance and grounding within constant change is the key to both happiness and beauty.

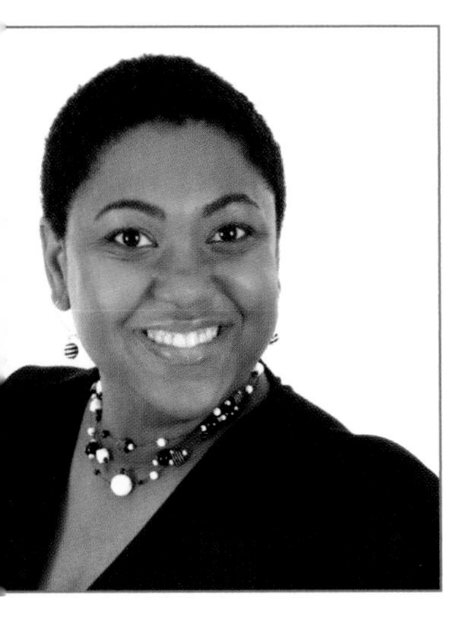

The Three Doshas:
Kapha, Pitta, Vata

Kapha:
Earth/ Water

Kapha is symbolized through water and earth. It represents growth, nutriments and their storage. Physically, Kaphas are slow-moving and fleshy with large, heavy-boned structures. Females are often voluptuous while males are inclined to be husky and to develop muscle easily. Their features are also full and substantial, their nails strong and hard. Kapha skin is thick and oily with a predisposition to enlarged pores, but if hydrated and healthy, their complexion can appear flawless. Kaphas are often considered classically beautiful as they possess large, radiant eyes, broad and prominent noses, full lips and luxuriant hair. Kaphas tend to be the healthiest, most robust of the doshas, as they have everything in abundance, including stamina and strong immune systems.

Their health problems also arise from that quality of abundance since Kaphas have a tendency to gain weight – a genetic trait reinforced by their habits. They may also suffer from sinus congestion (accumulation of mucous), edema (accumulation / retention of water), cystic acne (accumulation of toxins and oil).

Kaphas' physical qualities of heaviness, moistness, abundance and retention are reflected in their personalities. They are routine-oriented, grounded, nurturing, loyal and dependable. They have excellent knowledge-retention and are sentimental about holding onto tradition. They can also be incredibly romantic and sensuous lovers, since they understand the importance of taking time to enjoy each moment.

Kapha character flaws for Kaphas who are out of balance follow this same theme of abundance and retention. They are inclined toward greed, neediness and self-indulgence (accumulation of wealth, inability to let go, overeating, etc.) and can be resistant to change (lack of flexibility). Out of balance Kaphas (excess Kapha) may also be lethargic and depressive.

While Kapha bodies and temperaments are not often celebrated in our modern media, the Kapha ability to be still and stable is necessary to achieve the peace and serenity of Nirvana.

Pitta: Fire

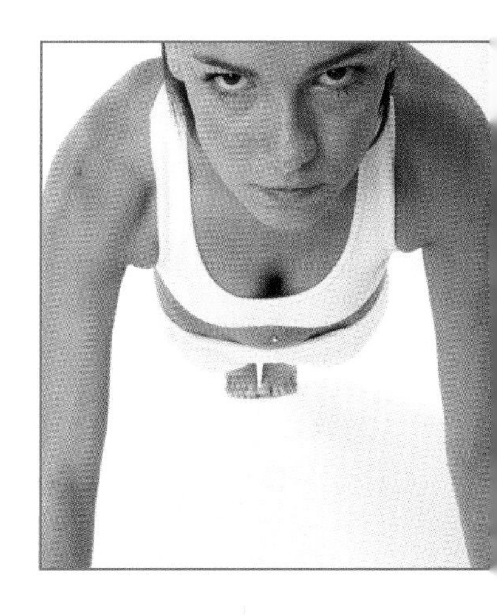

Pitta is represented by fire. Like fire, this dosha's qualities are hot, sharp and light. Pitta governs transformation, just as fire creates heat and heat causes chemical changes. It is the Pitta dosha that is responsible for transformations in the body through the metabolism (transforming storage to energy), digestion (transforming food to energy) and cellular transformation.

Physically, Pitta expresses itself in a medium, athletic build of average height. They embody heat with sensitive skin which can also be reactive. Pitta ailments stem from an excess of heat (fire) and acid. These include poor digestion, heartburn, allergies, acne, hyperacidity, rashes, hives, high blood pressure, dehydration, rosacea and liver disease. Because Pitta governs digestion, regular eating is very important to Pittas. When hungry, they become hot-headed, cranky and irritable.

Those with strong Pitta tend to be ambitious, competitive, well-organized and task-oriented. Because fire represents transformation, Pittas easily digest information, making them highly intelligent and conspicuous achievers. They are naturally charismatic, eloquent debaters, self-confident and passionate, all traits our society admires and rewards, which adds to their magnetism. Well-balanced Pittas make great leaders in business and in politics.

When out of balance, these fiery, Type A personalities can be opinionated, impatient, egotistical, uncompromising and overly-demanding to the point of being offensive. But through understanding Ayurveda, we can better understand that Pitta-predominant people are not difficult people, it is simply their nature to be the way they are. We can then appreciate their tendencies and avoid being hurt by their actions, accepting them with love. This transformation of perception is true for all three doshas, I simply find Pitta an easy example as they are easily seen as abrasive.

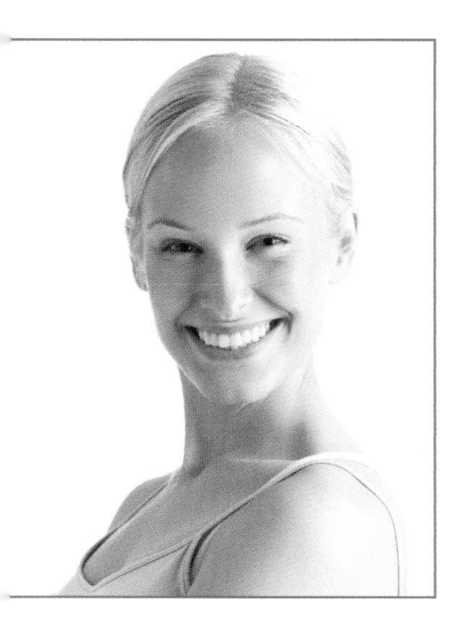

Vata:
Air/Ether

The Vata dosha embodies air. Like air, it is mobile, dry, rough and light. Vata, above all, governs movement. The circulation and the nervous systems are ruled by ever-changing Vata.

Vata-predominant people often seem more spirit than matter. Their willowy bodies are light and ethereal. Their skin is dry and thin, as well as rough and prone to fine-lines. Their nails are dry and brittle and their hair is also dry, fine and often curly. Along with their elongated silhouettes, Vatas have thin, chiseled features – sculpted cheekbones, long noses and thin lips.

Vata disorders relate to the nervous system, manifesting in such problems as paranoia, anxiety, worry and attention deficit disorder. Vatas' sensory organs are very acute, making them needful of harmony and easily disturbed by loud or jarring noises, crude images, objects rough to the touch and environmental chaos. They are also prone to kidney disease, bladder problems, low energy and excessive dryness.

The Vata personality is creative and excitable. Those dominated by this dosha are forward-thinkers, open-minded and flexible. They are early-adopters who desire innovation and new ideas, and who deeply appreciate beauty in design and art. Vatas love to learn, but often feel inadequate, unqualified, and unsure of their abilities despite their knowledge. Socially, they are adaptable and welcoming with excellent interpersonal skills. They also tend to be cerebral, ever-moving, ever-changing and unpredictable, making them both exciting and frustrating.

When in balance, Vatas are charming creatures, artistic, spiritual and entrepreneurial. When out-of-balance, they become paranoid, anxious, hyper, inconsistent, indecisive and in need of constant reassurance. Long term Vata-excess can make Vata dominant types unreliable, rash, impulsive and chaotic.

Physically delicate Vatas, with their elongated, graceful limbs and youthful energy, are today's poster-child of ideal beauty. But their true radiance is in their spiritualism and optimism.

Ayurveda and Contingency

Ayurveda is not a religion so much as a tool to better understand ourselves and others. Determining our dosha will also give us insight into our skin type, helping us to understand the root cause of any ailment and the best way to correct it. For example, Pitta acne is much different than Kapha acne, and Vata eczema must be treated differently than Pitta eczema. The reason they are different is because the cause is different, as I will explain in more detail in the acne and eczema sections of this book.

The concept of contingency is also fundamental to Ayurveda because the skin (along with the total body) is undergoing, and exposed to, constant change. Environment (weather, emotional states, diet) is just as important as classification. It is another version of nature vs. nurture, i.e. genetics vs. external forces.

Weather

Our skin behaves differently in different climates and seasons. Drier, colder conditions call for heavier, more nourishing skincare while warmer, wetter conditions need lighter products to let the skin breathe and absorb the moisture in the atmosphere. It is also important to change our skincare from day to day just as we change our clothing to suit the daily weather. A heavy moisturizing cream, like a winter coat, protects us from the elements while a lighter lotion, like a spring jacket, is better for warmer days.

The weather also affects the doshas resulting in changes within our bodies. Pitta increases when it is hot, causing fiery Pittas to get rashes, hives, inflammation and breakouts. They also exhibit Pitta's emotional characteristics, such as being short-tempered and irritable. Pittas feel most calm when pacified by cool weather.

Those with high Kapha will feel lethargic, heavy and puffy from water-retention during damp, cold and winter weather. They may also experience swollen eyes and excessive mucous. Kaphas are most in balance in hot, dry climates.

High Vata people will feel scattered, anxious and forgetful in windy, cool weather. Their skin will feel dry and flaky. Vatas function best when it is warm and humid.

Diet

Diet affects the nutritional environment of our skin. It is not only what you eat, but eating at appropriate times that gives the body and skin the nutrients to repair and protect itself. With diet, again the doshas exert their influence. High Pitta people should avoid hot, spicy and barbecued foods, especially when skin problems flare up; Kaphas should avoid heavy, creamy, fatty foods; Vatas should avoid dry, crunchy and astringent foods.

Time

As I have explained, everyone possesses all three doshas, usually with a predominance of one or two or the energies. But our constitution at birth is not the only factor which determines our energetic state, time also plays a part. During the course of a day, we respond to all three doshas because different doshic elements increase at different hours. Kapha is stronger in the morning (6 a.m.–10 a.m.) and early evening (6 p.m.–10 p.m.), while Pitta is strongest between the hours of 10 a.m. and 2 p.m. and 10 p.m and 2 a.m. Vata time is from 2 a.m to 6 a.m. and 2 p.m. and 6 p.m., and is strongest during hours of transition (dawn and dusk). This demonstrates why waking up early invigorates us (we clear Kapha drowsiness); why eating our largest meal at lunch is best for digestion (Pitta is ignited), and why we suffer from insomnia if we do not go to bed early enough (Vata is awakened in the body during the late hours).

Menstrual Cycle

For women, menses affect many aspects of the skin – most commonly in the form of break outs and sensitivity. The doshas fluctuate throughout our menstrual cycle as Kapha is high between the end of our menstrual flow and ovulation (Kapha prepares the womb), Pitta is high from ovulation until flow begins (when Pitta is in excess, it is exhibited through PMS) and Vata is high during the days of flow (Vata governs movement). This greatly affects our physical and emotional bodies.

Emotional States

How we think and feel impacts our bodies more than most of us realize. Stress dehydrates the skin, and eczema can be triggered by post-traumatic stress disorder. Because the doshas govern different emotions, an imbalance in the doshas will also wreak havoc on our emotional wellbeing. The opposite is also true. When we experience emotional disruption, this will affect the state of the doshas within our bodies. In some ways, the emotional factor is harder to treat; in other ways it makes things easier because once we identify the issue as it is within our power to resolve it.

The Doshas and the Stages of Life

Self-diagnosing can often be difficult. When I encountered Ayurveda in my mid-teens, I thought I was a Pitta-Kapha because I displayed strong Kapha characteristics. I was lethargic, I had an intolerance to wet, mucous-forming foods (milk, heavy starches, etc.), and I was resistant to change. When properly diagnosed by Dr. Vasant Lad, I was surprised to find that I was a Pitta-Vata. My Kapha afflictions were partly due to a Kapha imbalance which was emphasized as I was in the Kapha stage of life. This heightened these characteristics.

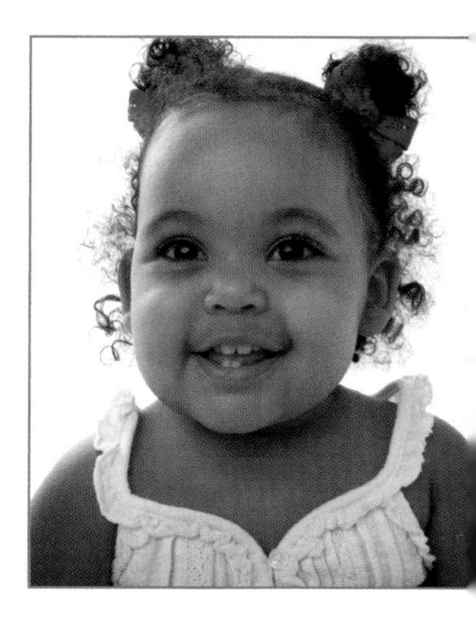

Kapha: Our growth years

Kapha is strongest during our formative years, from birth through our teens and into our early twenties. This is when we are growing physically and accumulating knowledge. We have baby fat and our skin is as moist as it will ever be. We are self-centered, self-indulgent, and our memory is at its best.

This is also the time when many children experience wet eczema and excessive mucous from allergies, while teens experience wet acne. Avoiding moist, Kapha-forming foods (dairy products, sweet and salty foods, starches) helps alleviate these ailments.

Kapha also loves to sleep in, which aggravates their problems, while rising early helps eliminate them. Cardiovascular exercise is also recommended, since stimulation is the key to clearing excess Kapha.

Ayurveda prescribes a vigorous massage using powder instead of oil to promote circulation. Through the traction of the powder, fatty tissue is mobilized and Kapha stagnation is stimulated.

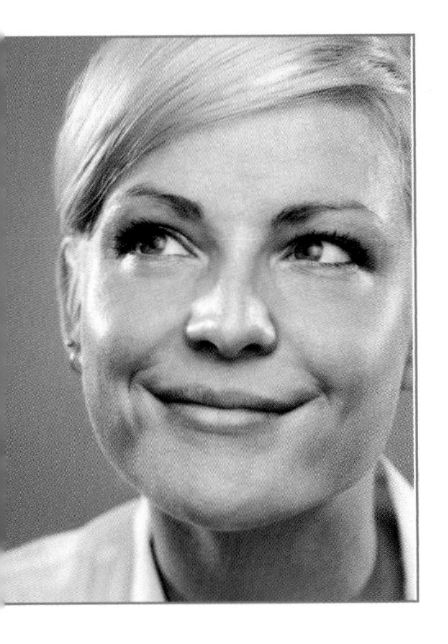

Pitta:
A time of action

The twenties through the forties are our Pitta years. This is when our lives are action-oriented and career-focused. Excess Pitta is caused by overly-ambitious expectations and by pushing our bodies too hard. This sometimes leads to a compromised liver and an adverse reaction to foods. It is also the time when rosacea (known as adult acne) is most aggravated, along with broken capillaries and uneven pigmentation.

Avoiding overheated, overcooked, spicy foods helps soothe Pitta excesses, as does cooler temperatures. Unfortunately, Pitta loves hard exercise, which creates more heat. Yogic practices and meditation help balance out the body's fire, as well as calming and clearing the mind. Pittas cannot take heavy oils as they increase heat, but lightweight oils such as coconut and jojoba are great for cooling the skin. Saunas should be avoided.

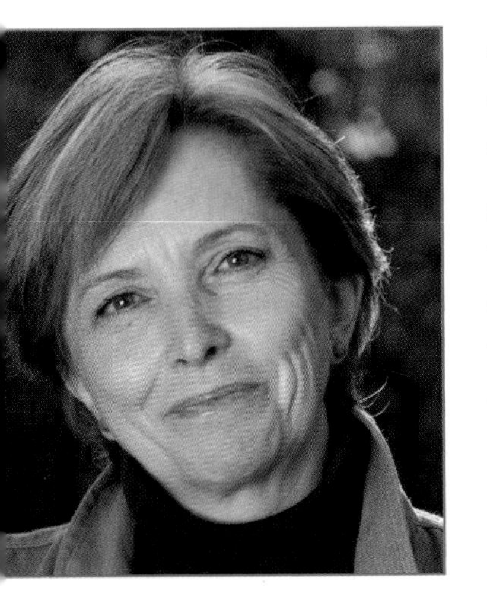

Vata:
Era of the spirit

Vata becomes very influential as we move into maturity. We grow more spiritual as we approach the end of our lives, but though we may have gained in wisdom, we have likely decreased in matter. With a decline in collagen production, we lose weight and decrease in height. Our skin becomes drier, wrinkled, crinkled and thinned. Our thoughts may become more scattered, like air, while memories escape us.

Promoting Kapha is beneficial as a countermeasure, and persons with strong Kapha seem to age the best. Eating moist, heavy foods and getting ample sleep is beneficial in minimizing Vata-excess. Daily massaging of the body and scalp with sesame oil is also excellent. Vatas, in particular, should get a regular, relaxing massage with heavy, nourishing oils. Absorbing these through the skin's nerve endings pacifies Vata, and counters the over-activity of their nervous system.

While Kapha combats aging caused by an excess of Pitta and Vata, it is said that Pitta and Vata doshas are the energies which ascend the soul to the next realm. Though our youth-obsessed culture encourages us to fight the aging process, beauty can also come from letting nature take its course.

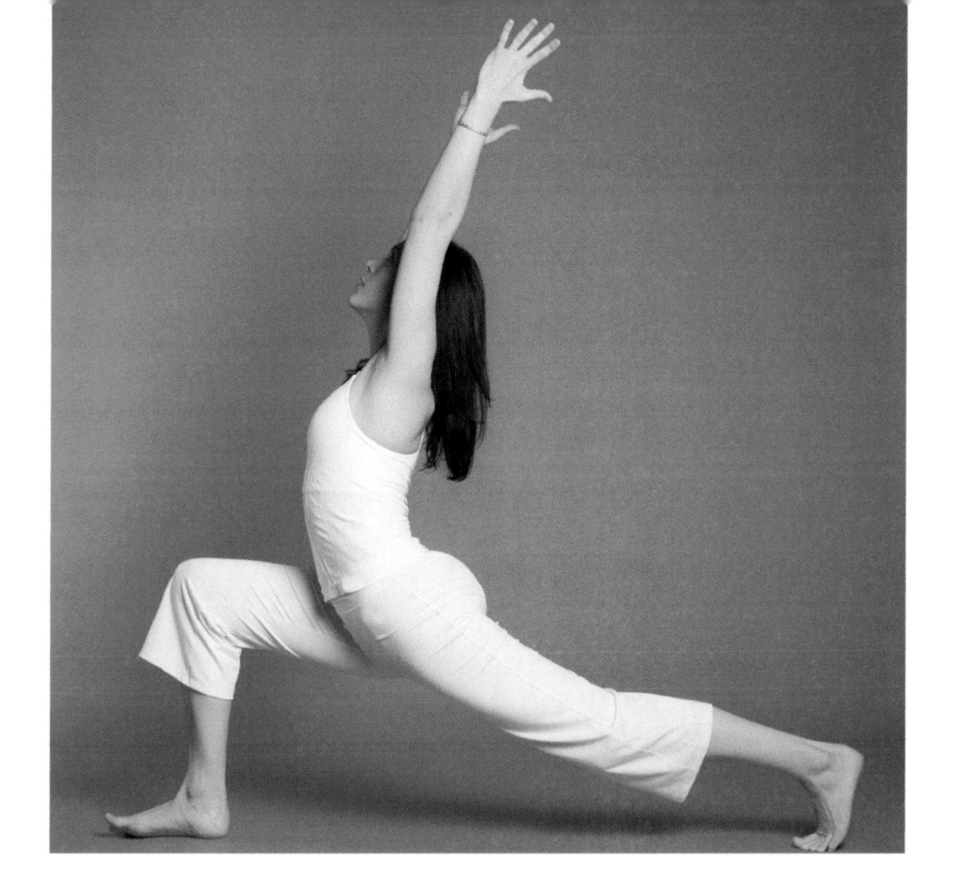

Ayurvedic Anti-aging

Rasayana, a branch of Ayurvedic medicine, is a method of regeneration. It is used after any detoxification or surgical procedure, and as a preventative tool for overall wellbeing. Ayurveda does not believe in cleansing or removing damaged tissue without replenishing and nourishing to avoid a relapse.

Ayurveda defines aging as the time when the body has greater tissue loss than tissue gain. This is due to increased Vata (depletion of matter) and the accumulation of metabolic waste which inhibits cellular regeneration (tissue gain).

Panchakarma, which is a program of detoxification, is said to be necessary to maintain youthful vibrancy. This coupled with Rasayana therapy ensures the health of our tissues as Panchakarma removes waste and Rasayana supports the body's replenishment.

Rasayana herbs are packed with antioxidants and help promote cellular growth. Though Ayurveda advocates herbs, like shatavari, ashwaghanda or guduchi to nurture the tissue and the soul, other regenerating herbs and treatments from other modalities can be just as effective. It is the role of healing which makes Rasayana important.

Ayurvedic Mind – Body Constitution Questionnaire

1. Sensitive to	A. Dry, cold, windy	B. Heat and Sun	C. Cold and Damp
2. Skin	A. Dry, thin, rough	B. Combination, Sensitive, Pigmentation	C. Oily, Moist, Thick
3. Pores	A. Small, Fine	B. Large in T-zone	C. Large, Open
4. Complexion	A. Fine lines, Sallow	B. Redness, Broken Capillaries, Moles, Freckles, Rosacea	C. Blackheads, Excess oiliness. If Uncongested: Soft, Youthful, Clear
5. Skin Ailments	A. Dehydration A. Excessive Dryness A. Dry Eczema A. Psoriasis A. Cracked Skin A. Under-eye Circles	B. Inflammation B. Acne Rosacea B. Burning Eczema B. Rash, Hives B. Infected Blemishes B. Contact Dermatitis	C. Dullness C. Water Retention C. Wet/Itchy Eczema C. Loss of Tone/Jowls C. Cystic Acne
6. Facial features	A. Chiseled, Fine, Long, Oval A. Thin, Dry, Irregular Lips	B. Medium Proportions B. Sharp, Piercing eyes	C. Large, Round or Square with Soft Contours C. Large Eyes C. Thick, Soft, Even Lips
7. Hair	A. Dry, Thin, Coarse, Curly, Wiry	B. Red Tones, Straight, Premature Greying or Balding	C. Thick, Oily, Wavy, Abundant
8. Fingernails	A. Dry, Weak, Brittle, Discoloured, Irregular,	B. Soft, Medium, Pink	C. Strong, Smooth, Regular Shaped Cuticles
9. Physical Build	A. Thin, Tall, Long-Limbed	B. Average with Good Muscle Tone	C. Voluptuous,Husky, Prone to Overweight
10. Physical Activity	A. Active, Quick with Low Endurance	B. Athletic, Average Strength, Intolerant to Heat	C. Lethargic, Slow to Start with Good Endurance
11. Mental Activity	A. Restless, Erratic, Creative, Chaotic A. Quick to Learn but Poor Memory	B. Focused, Goal-driven B. Strong Memory	C. Calm, Steady, Cautious C. Slow to Grasp but Good Memory
12. Temperament	A. Insecure, Unpredictable, Excitable	B. Aggressive, Irritable, Impatient, Jealous	C. Calm, Sentimental, Prone to Depression
13. Ailments	A. Kidney Problems A. Constipation A. Bloating/ Gas A. Arthritis A. Weight Loss A. Low Appetite	B. High Acid B. Liver Disease B. Hypertension B. Inflammatory Disease B. Hemorrhoids	C. Sinus Congestion C. Asthma C. Bronchitis C. Obesity C. High Cholesterol C. Drowsiness

14. Menses	A. Irregular, Scanty Flow, Severe Cramps	B. May Have Heavy Bleeding	C. Prone to Water Retention, Slight Cramps
15. Diet	A. Either Indulges or Strict Diet	B. Loves Protein, Caffeine, Spicy, Salty Foods	C. Loves Sweets, Dairy, Carbs
16. Gums	A. Receding Gums	B. Inflamed Gums	C. Thick Gums
17. Joints	A. Pain in Joints, Stiff, Cracking, Unsteady	B. Hot, Burning	C. Aching, Swollen, Watery
18. Decision-Making	A. Indecisive A. Quick to Change Mind/ View	B. Rapid Decision-Making	C. Takes Time to Decide
19. Thinking Style	A. Creative Thinker	B. Organized Thinker	C. Conservative Thinker
20. Mental Activity	A. Restless, Active	B. Aggressive, Likes Competition	C. Calm, Likes to Relax
21. Approach to Change	A. Seeks Change	B. Plans and Proceeds in an Organized Fashion	C. Resists Change, Likes Simplicity
22. Relationships	A. Very Social, Knows Many People A. Very Few Close Friends	B. Very Selective B. Needs Attention B. Makes Enemies Easily	C. Few Friends, but Very Close C. Loyal C. Sentimental
23. Spending Habits	A. Spends Impulsively	B. Spends to Achieve a Purpose B. Spends on Luxury Goods	C. Likes to Save C. Spends Reluctantly
24. Roles	A. Conceptualizes	B. Executes	C. Maintains
25. Experiences and Traits	A. Fear A. Nervous A. Anxious A. Non-Committal A. Youthful A. Flexible A. Receptive	B. Anger B. Judgmental B. Impatient B. Egotistical B. Instrumental B. Controlling B. Opinionated	C. Depression C. Apathetic C. Patient C. Self-Indulgent C. Maternal C. Inflexible C. Resists Giving
26. Conflict Resolution	A. Accommodating	B. Insistent	C. Passive
Answer key:	**Mostly A: Vata**	**Mostly B: Pitta**	**Mostly C: Kapha.**

The ratios of A:B:C indicate the ratios of each dosha within our constitution. This test is a basic guide, but the most accurate diagnosis will come from a professional/ practitioner who can analyze pulse, history and other physical indicators.

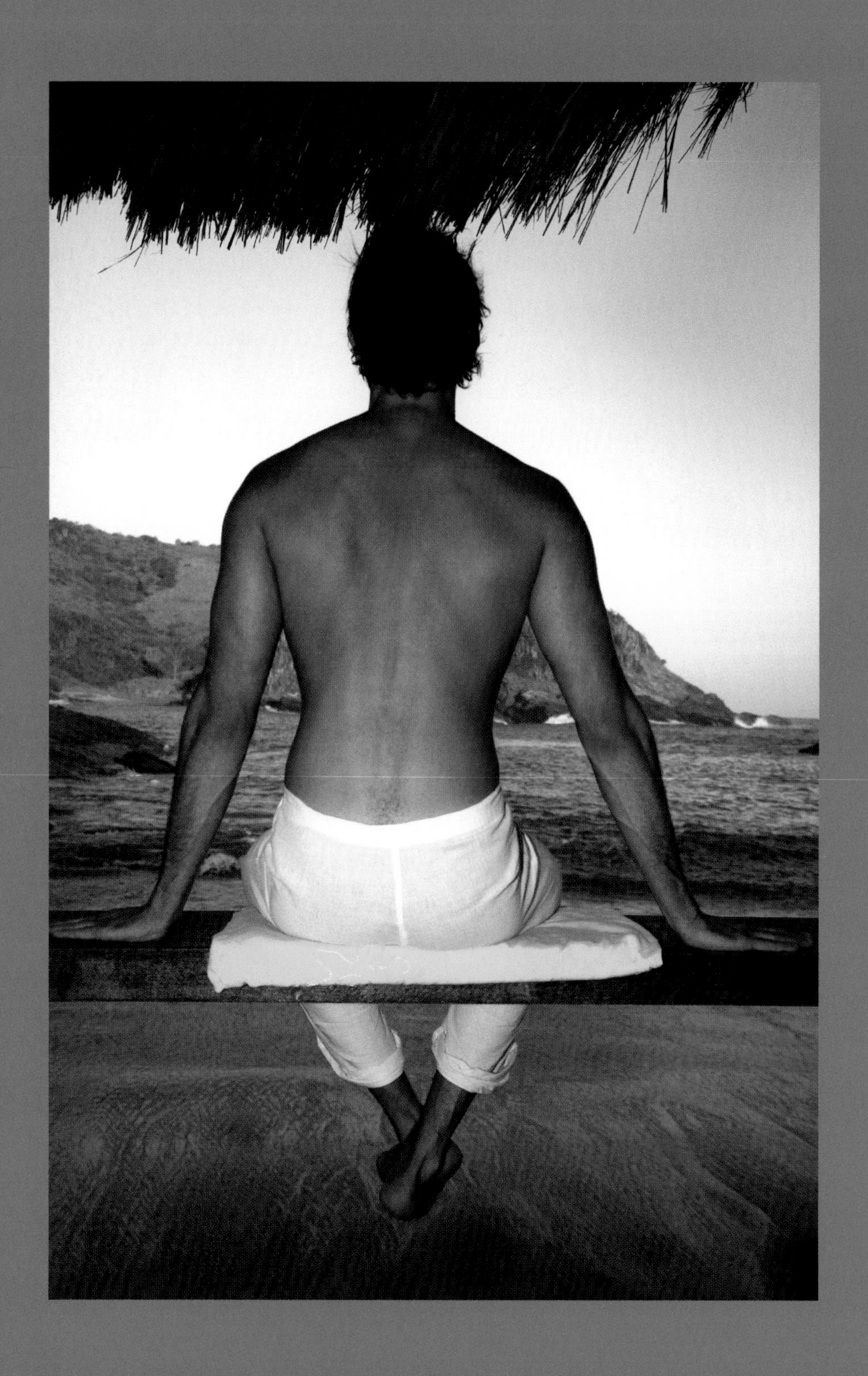

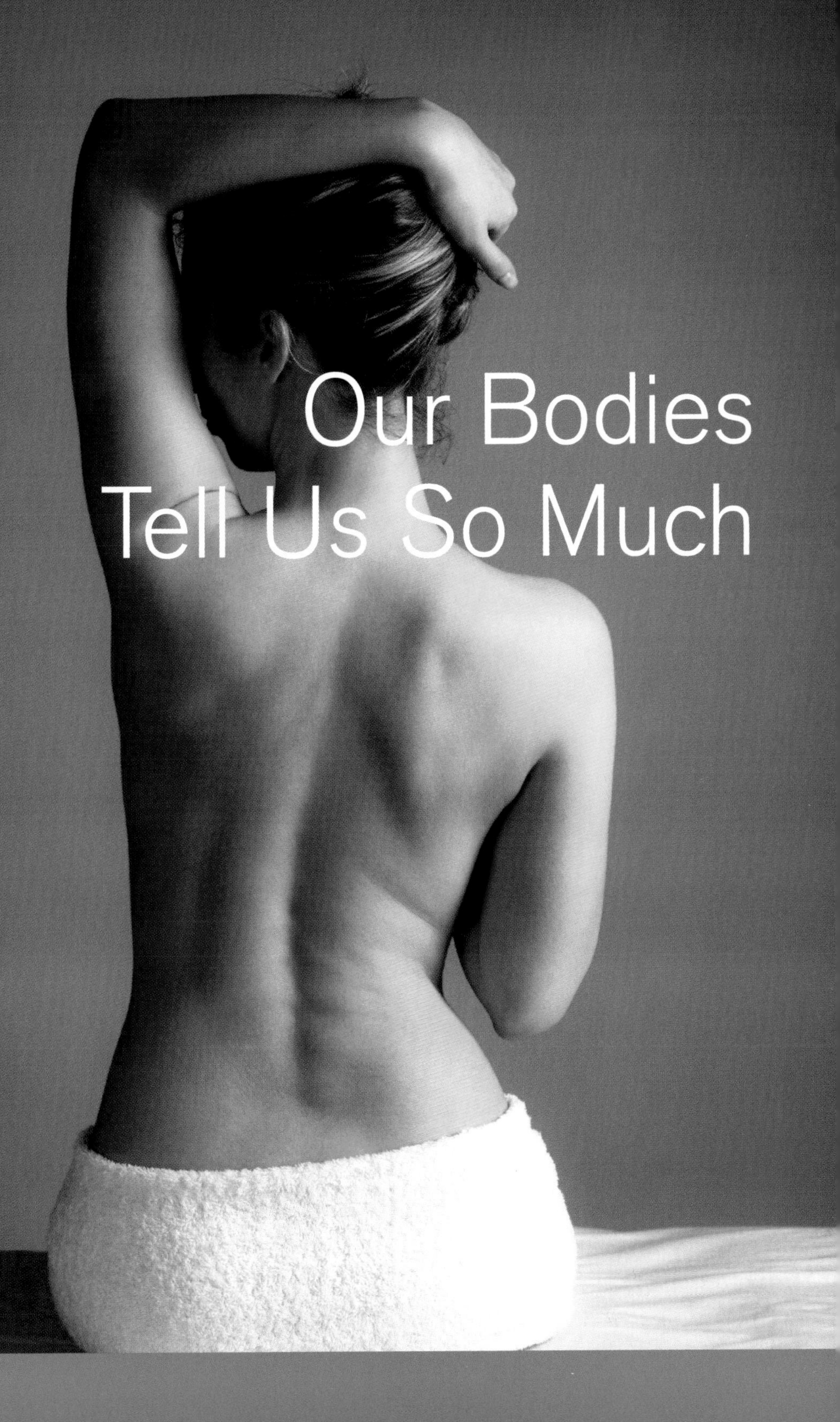

Our Bodies Tell Us So Much

CHAPTER 4

Our bodies tell us so much...

Examining the skin is a wonderful way to see how the body communicates the state of our internal health through the external body.

While facial blemishes and wrinkles may appear unsightly, they help us to monitor the internal body. Dermatologists and Beauty Consultants often prescribe harsh creams to camouflage these skin imperfections, whereas traditional Eastern Practitioners use them as a guide to "read" our organs. This is called face-mapping.

Ayurvedic Doshas and the Parts of the Face

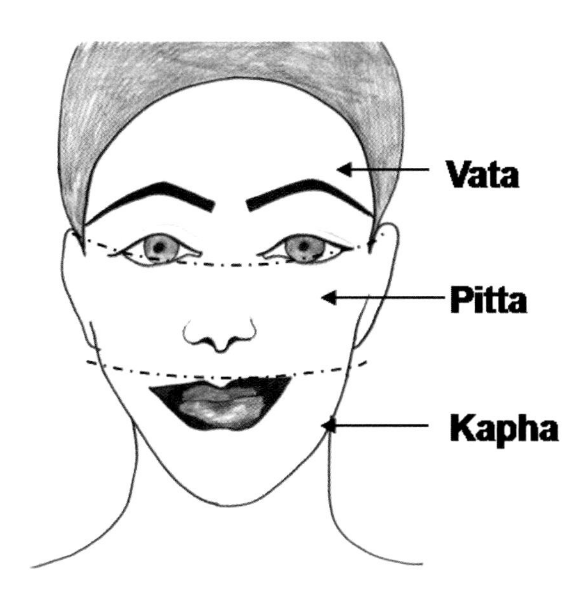

In Ayurveda, each dosha governs different sections of the face, different organs and different body parts. While this makes for a very complex ideology, it produces a simple guide for skincare.

Vata governs the upper section of the face above the eyes. Pitta governs the middle section between the eyes and the mouth. Kapha governs the lower face. Skin ailments affecting these areas are often due to an imbalance of the corresponding dosha.

Vata: Forehead

The forehead, which is the thinnest and driest area of the face, is where the Vata expresses itself. Worry lines here are caused by anxiety and fear. Vata emotions also produce insomnia and other stress-related disorders which contribute further to worry lines.

Many people also have congestion isolated to the forehead, which is often linked to constipation, as the colon is governed by Vata. When treating such people for skin dehydration, it is also necessary to detoxify the colon and to calm the mind.

Pitta: Cheeks and Nose

Pitta rules the centre of the face, where rosacea, whiteheads and broken capillaries are often found. Rosacea is a cardiovascular disorder caused by anger, jealousy, and stress from pressure to succeed (this usually is self-inflicted since Pittas are highly ambitious).

Teenagers often have red, blistering acne in this area caused by the hormonal heat of puberty. Acne restricted to the cheeks or nose should be treated with cooling herbs, blood purification and detoxification of the small intestine.

Smoking also increases internal heat. The stopping of smoking will help lessen both signs of rosacea and irritated break outs in this section of the face.

Kapha: Lower Cheeks, Jaw, Lips and Chin

The lower face is governed by Kapha. An imbalance here may manifest as a double chin (excess fat) caused by hypothyroidism. Cystic acne, with Kapha qualities of fluid-retention and fullness, is most commonly found on the chin and jaw line. These types of deep-seated blemishes are also caused by hormonal imbalances.

The Kapha area often breaks out in cysts because of internal toxin-retention, as well as stagnation of the lymphatic fluid (holding on and accumulation). It can also reflect lethargy, emotional repression or an inability to let go.

Treat acne in the Kapha region with lymphatic stimulation and a Kapha-reducing diet low in sweets, salt, oily and fatty foods.

Beauty and the Organs

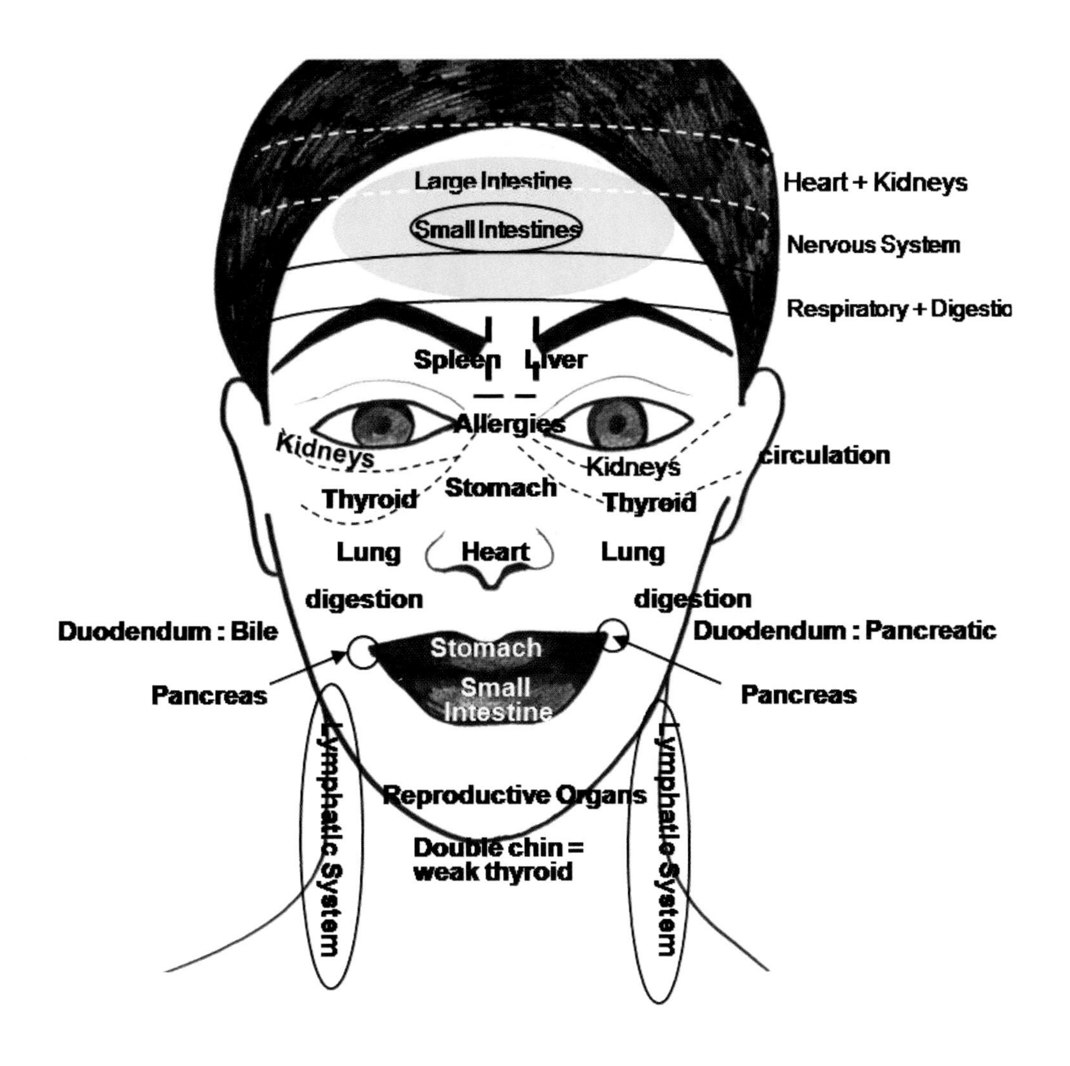

CHINESE FACE MAP

For a more detailed reading of this face map as the cause of skin conditions, I would like to refer to the following sections on *Beauty and the Organs* as well as *The Connection Between the Organs.* TCM practitioners generally accept the subsequent correlations.

Beauty and the Organs

In TCM, just as in Ayurveda, our organs relate to other tissues and body parts in specific ways. It is fascinating to see how ancient practitioners saw these interactions, and also how external imperfections reflect what is going on inside the body.

Under-Eye Circles: Weak Kidneys

If the kidneys are being overtaxed, this will also interfere with sleep and further contribute to dark circles. Decreasing salt-intake, ensuring regular water-intake, limiting protein consumption and proper rest will all help restore the kidneys.

Frown Lines between the Eyebrows: Overworked Liver and Spleen

The wrinkles perpendicular to the right brow relate to the liver; the ones to the left, to the spleen. To detoxify an overtaxed liver, start by eating leafy greens supplemented with a milk-thistle tincture. Treating these superficially with Botox injections simply adds toxins to the body.

Dry Lips: Dehydrated Stomach and Small Intestines

The lips relate to the digestive organs – the upper lip to the stomach, the lower one to the small intestine. Most often, applying lip balm is not sufficient. We must hydrate our bodies, making sure no dry stool is left in our intestines, further drying out the body. Colonics and enemas can assist this. While colonics (colon irrigation) insert water into the colon through the anus to alleviate constipation, Ayurveda advocates medicated enemas (called Bastis) as they are said to be less abrasive. Bastis can use oils or herbal infusions to loosen dry stool while healing the intestinal wall.

Upper Lip Wrinkles: Sexual Debility

This area relates to the sex organs. Wrinkles here show a dysfunction with the reproductive organs, such as sterility and sexual debility. Chain smokers develop wrinkles here because cigarette smoking can damage the sex organs. Ayurveda prescribes taking Shatavari to cleanse and regenerate the reproductive organs but every school of thought has its own herbs for this function.

Red Nose: Stress on the Heart

This is the Pitta area, signifying an overworked heart and high blood pressure. Alcoholics often acquire redness and broken capillaries because alcohol is heating. Cleansing the blood and strengthening the heart is important. Neem and Burdock root are examples of herbs that help with this.

The Connections Between the Organs

It is also important to note how interconnected our systems are. Each organ relates to others, and its health dictates the state of these other organs. As our organs dictate the healthiness of our tissues, this will also affect our physical appearance.

The Heart:

The heart relates to the small intestine and is in charge of capillaries. It is also part of the mind and is reflected in the face. When we are stressed or weighed down emotionally, our heart is greatly taxed, affecting our complexion. Rosacea is the perfect example of how the skin relates to the heart through stressed capillaries.

The Lungs:

According to TCM, the lungs relate to the colon and open through the nose. The state of the lungs is reflected in the skin and body hair. The skin, the lungs and the colon are all channels of elimination, which is why allergic reactions often occur here. If the lungs are taxed with allergies or respiratory problems, this will also be displayed in the quality and texture of our skin and hair.

Zang (yin) organs:
Organs which have substance and are not hollow. Lung, liver, spleen, kidneys, heart, pericardium (heart lining).

Fu (yang) organs:
Organs which are empty and which are emptied (hollow, expanding organs which are bag-like and involve much action). Small and large intestines, gallbladder, stomach, bladder, triple warmer (the muscle casing containing other organs in the trunk of the body).

The Spleen:

The spleen relates to the stomach, opens through the mouth and limbs, and is reflected in the lips. As mentioned before, the stomach and small intestine dictate dry lips, but sometimes lips are so dry that they are puffy with water-retention as the spleen plays a role in water-metabolism.

The Liver:

The liver relates to the gallbladder, opens into the eyes and is reflected in the nails. Strong, beautiful nails are indicative of a healthy liver and gallbladder. Weak, breaking or nicked nails indicate a weak immune system or malnourishment. This is because the liver is the filtration system of the body and the gallbladder assists digestion.

The Kidneys:

The kidneys relate to the bladder, and open through the ears and the lower orifices. They are in charge of bones and reflected in the hair of the head. As we grow older, our kidneys and our bones become weaker. Arthritis is very much connected to the kidneys. Hair loss is also related to weak kidneys and stress affects the kidneys, which is why stress plays a role in balding. Strengthening the kidneys and calming Vata will restore the hair, strengthen bones and pacify arthritis.

Caring for the Internal Body

Given the relationship between the skin and the organs, it is obvious that skin ailments communicate what needs to be healed within our bodies. This also demonstrates that no skin problem can be totally cured without reference to lifestyle and total body health.

When I had acne as a teenager, many doctors and estheticians told me that my blemishes had nothing to do with my diet or my general physical and emotional state; however, until these were addressed, I saw no changes in my skin. While professionals may now, more or less, accept these factors, I do not think many understand how significant they are.

Examples of how our body's health can affect our emotions:

- An overwhelmed liver can cause excessive anger.
- A weak kidney can breed fear and worry.
- A toxic colon can induce depression.

Examples of how our internal health affects the external body:

- Acne is often caused by the body's purging of toxins from the liver (excessive yang rising).
- Overworked kidneys can cause dehydrated skin because kidneys regulate our body's water.
- A food allergy often manifests through rashes, redness or itchiness.
- As the body ages, the skin's appearance changes. Prolonged illness can cause the skin to appear dull, yellow or blue.
- A cardiovascular disorder can result in rosacea.

The Skin as an Indicator of the Body's Needs

The skin is an excellent barometer of our health. When the body lacks water, the skin will be the first organ forced to dehydrate, allowing us to quickly identify and balance the situation. The solution can be as easy as applying more moisturizer, drinking more fluids and eating less meat. In more extreme cases, herbs are required to detoxify the kidneys, and the adrenals need to be supported and rejuvenated.

When our elimination system is insufficient to detoxify the body, toxins will be eliminated through the skin. Purifying the skin topically is only a start. Giving the digestive system a rest so it can detoxify is another good immediate response. Herbs can also help cleanse our colon and kidneys (organs of elimination) as well as our liver (our organ of filtration). A more in-depth program would involve making sure we have one to two daily bowel movements, nourishing our body with vitamins, minerals and oxygen (for prana), and promoting better circulation.

Acne and Elimination

The most obvious example of poor elimination is acne. Acne in adults is usually liver-related, unlike teenage acne which is more often caused by hormonal imbalances. While teenage acne can also be liver-related, the toxic buildup is not the same as for adults. Despite being unsightly, acne may not be such a bad thing, since it indicates our bodies are purging toxins rather than holding them where they could lead to more serious damage.

Ironically, a popular solution for acne is to take antibiotics which dry out our internal organs, and make us photosensitive (vulnerable to the sun). Hydration is imperative for waste elimination. Like a dried up river, our system cannot flow and flush itself. Even facial purging in the form of extractions is hard to achieve when our skin is dried out. Obviously, these drugs are not a healthy, long-term solution.

Bowels and Elimination

Our bowels are our first avenue of elimination. While we may feel we are eliminating regularly, many people do not properly realize that we should be having bowel movements twice per day ideally. If waste is not purged from our body, toxins accumulate, causing illness and inflammation.

Our bowels must be cleansed before any other organ. While it is also important to detoxify the liver, kidneys, gallbladder, etc., if the bowels are backed up, other detoxification is impossible. Colonic irrigation and enemas have been previously mentioned to cleanse the bowels deeply. I have seen much success in all areas of health when these therapies are employed, but we must also be wary over-stimulating the colon. Frequent colonics can be irritating to the large intestine, so I would advise having a practitioner outline a series of treatments that take care of individual needs in a conscious way.

The Liver: Our Filtration System

The liver, governed by Pitta, is the body's filtration system and is central to the elimination of waste in our body. It also regulates our hormones. When our bowels are not functioning properly, waste overloads the liver until it cannot function properly either. It becomes like a wet sponge which cannot absorb or filter anything more. Toxins will overspill into other organs, to be purged through the skin or the lungs (through coughing up mucous).

Liver Cleansing Herbs:

- Milk thistle
- Neem
- Dandelion

Inflamed Skin and Elimination

Reactive skin (allergy-prone) is also due to toxicity. In Ayurveda, it is called ama. We react to our external environment when our bodies are so overtaxed by inner toxins that they cannot handle external stimulants. Rosacea is caused by inflammation which, in turn, is a response to toxins (Pitta ama). Similarly, when the lymphs are full and in need of draining, they create pressure which dilates and breaks our capillaries.

Eczema and psoriasis also indicate a need for detoxification. While these conditions are often stress-triggered, toxins actually create the sensitivity.

Remember the principles of Ayurveda – no food or therapy is a universal good. Each person and each dosha responds to different things. For instance, laxatives: Vatas are so dry that psyllium constipates them, while Kaphas have the moisture for it. Vatas do better with moist laxatives such as soaked prunes, mangos and castor oil. Pittas respond well to cooling laxatives such as aloe vera juice.

Herbs and foods for healthy digestion and bowels:

- Healthy intestinal flora: Probiotics
- Purgatives (laxatives): aloe vera, castor oil, flax seed oil, triphala, prunes,
- Scraping the intestinal wall: fibre, honey

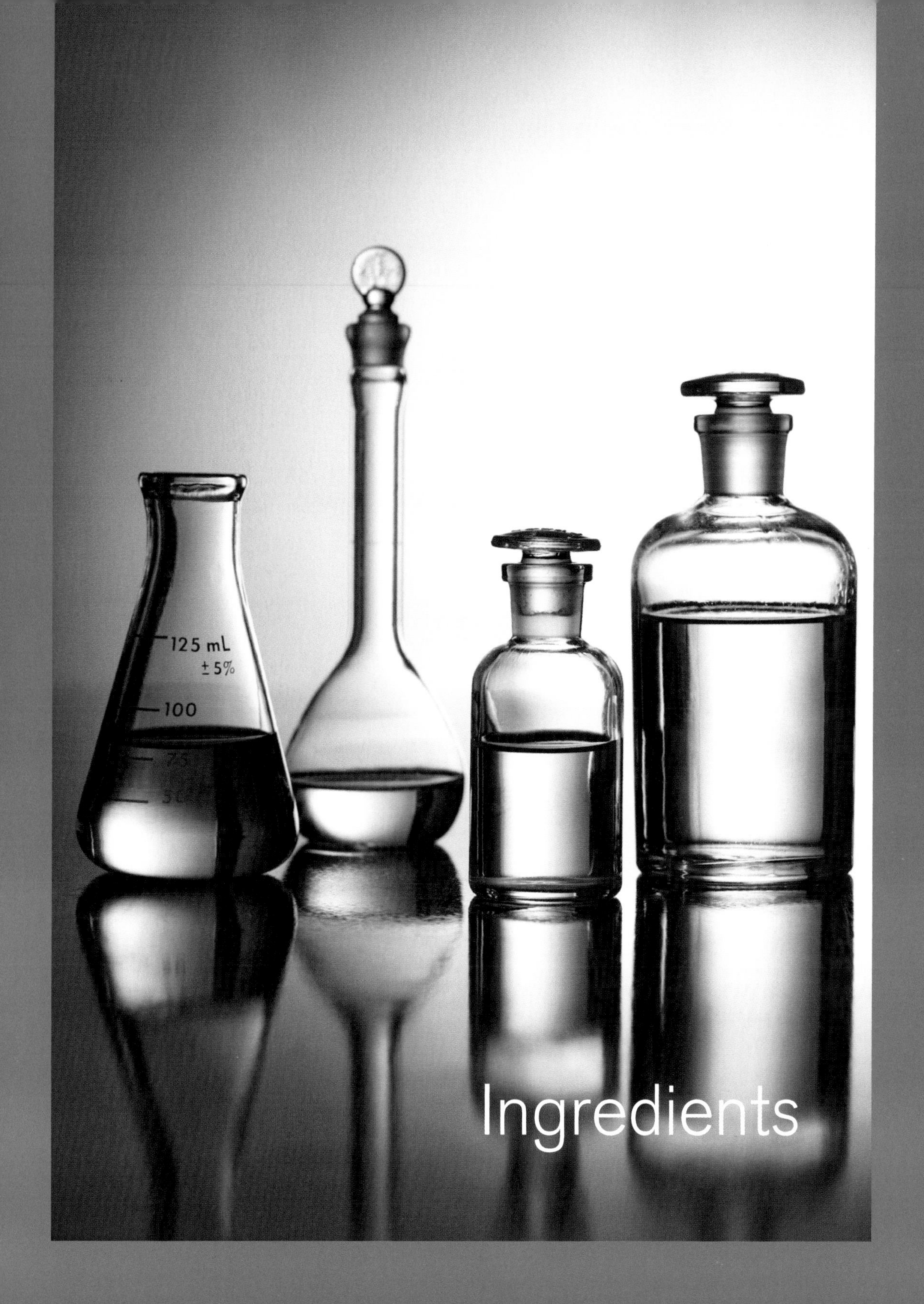

Ingredients

CHAPTER 5

Ingredients to Avoid
For healthy bodies and complexions

Two Common Ingredients to Avoid

Despite an abundance of information about the benefits of natural cosmetics and the dangers of many toxic chemicals, some of the latter are still widely used in skin-care and other grooming products. Here are two of the worst and most important to avoid:

1. Petrolatum/ Paraffinium Liquidum

Function: Petroleum is primarily used as a cosmetic base.
Found in: Almost all cosmetics, skincare and hair products.
Also known as: Mineral Oil, Petroleum. There are many more names.
Derivation: Petroleum By-Product

Causes Pore-congestion

When we check to see what is in our mysterious bottles of skincare goop, we find it is mainly petroleum, a few additives and a lot of water. The problem with petroleum/paraffinium is that its molecules are too large to fully penetrate the skin. Therefore, products made with it sit on the skin's surface clogging its pores. In the early years of my career, working at one of the most elite but conventional spas in Sydney, Australia, I ran out of the petroleum jelly we used to protect the delicate skin around the eyes from dye while doing a lash tint. I was told to substitute it with a very expensive brand of neck cream. That was when I realized this high-end neck cream was simply fancied up petroleum jelly. It was appropriate to use because it would sit on the skin and act as a barrier.

Petroleum dehydrates the skin, which is ironic, since it is used as the base for most moisturizers. Though many of these feature wonderful ingredients (antioxidants, vitamins, etc.) they cannot be fully absorbed into the skin. I often compare using petroleum on the skin to masking the face with saran wrap. While it makes an excellent barrier for acute situations (against windburn while skiing etc.), it is unhealthy when used on a daily basis.

Many people – myself included – find they self-induce acne through petroleum-based products. The pore build-up contributes to comedones and blemishes. These products can also irritate sensitive skin and trigger allergies.

Another example of petroleum as a barrier is antiperspirant. In addition to containing aluminum, antiperspirant sticks are petroleum-based, inhibiting the sudoriferous (sweat) glands.

The Internal Damage

Petroleum also has its dangers internally. While much of it sits on the skin, what little absorbs has been found to cause kidney damage and liver abnormalities. It is the same material as petrol, or gasoline, and we are applying it on our faces, bodies and scalps.

Besides the direct harm to our bodies, petrochemicals take vast amounts of energy to produce and are nonrenewable.

2. Sodium Laurel Sulfate

Function: A cleansing and foaming agent

Found in: Cleansers, shampoos, soaps, toothpaste, astringent, toners

Also called: SLS

Strips the Skin

Sodium laurel sulfate is a harsh detergent mostly found in products whose function is to clean. It has a foaming property and gives the skin that tight feeling many perceive as being "deeply cleansed." In fact, SLS disturbs the skin's acid mantle and strips it of its natural oils. This is especially detrimental for sensitive skins, leading to rosacea, eczema and dermatitis.

The body is always working to attain balance and to heal. It has awesome regenerative powers, which extend to the skin. When we use SLS products, the body attempts to balance out the dryness it creates by producing more oil; therefore, while SLS dehydrates aging skin, it stimulates oil production in oily skin. The now-overactive sebaceous glands pour out sebum (oil) to compensate for the skin's dehydration.

The Internal Damage

SLS is absorbed and then retained in the eyes, brain, heart, liver and other organs. It is also absorbed into the delicate mouth tissues via toothpaste and into the scalp via shampoos and conditioners. Having stripped the skin of its defenses, it increases the absorption of other toxic materials, making us more vulnerable to disease. Studies have also shown that sodium laurel sulfate combines with various cosmetic ingredients to create carcinogenic nitrates and dioxin. It is thought to retard healing and promote tissue malformation.

Other ingredients to avoid

Propylene and Butylene glycol

These are petroleum-derived ingredients used in skin and hair products to temporarily boost skin hydration. Long-term, they can dehydrate and damage the skin's structure. Refer back to the "Petrolatum/ Paraffinium Liquidum" section for effects on our internal bodies.

Carbomer

A petroleum-derived thickener, carbomer masks the fact that a product may be mostly composed of water and not of skin-nourishing ingredients. Used commonly in creams, bath products and eye makeup.

Sunscreening agents

Some chemical sunscreen agents, like benzophenone and octy-methoxycinnamate, mimic estrogen, confusing our endocrine system. In contrast, mineral sunblocks, like zinc oxide and titanium, are natural materials that reduce photo-activity.

Parabens (butyl- ethyl- methyl- and propyl-)

These parabens are a formaldehyde-derived group of preservatives for cosmetics and food. They mimic estrogen and have been cited as carcinogens.

Cortisone

Cortisone is a steroid used for its anti-inflammatory effects. Long term, it thins the skin and weakens its immune response. Internally, it is also known to suppress immune response. Cortisone creams are often prescribed by dermatologists to soothe eczema, acne and general inflammation.

Phlalates

A group of liquid chemicals, resembling oil, phlalates serve as a fixative to slow evaporation, causing the scent in perfumes and other products to linger. They are also used as a plasticizer in nail polish. Phlalates are endocrine disrupters and carcinogenic. They are said to cause blood-clotting, along with damage to the heart and lungs.

Coal tar

Used to manufacture commercial dyes and industrial paints, coal tar is also an ingredient in colour cosmetics, hair dyes and makeup. It is known to be a carcinogen and a photo-sensitizer.

Diethanolamine (DEA)

Diethanolamine is a chemical used as a wetting agent and to give texture to lotions and creams, as well as a foaming agent in shampoos and body washes. It becomes unsafe when it reacts with the product's other ingredients, possibly turning into a hormone-disruptor and a carcinogen.

Diazolidinyl urea, Imidazolidinyl urea

These are common preservatives for cosmetics that release formaldehyde. They are known carcinogens and trigger allergies. They can also cause contact dermatitis and headaches.

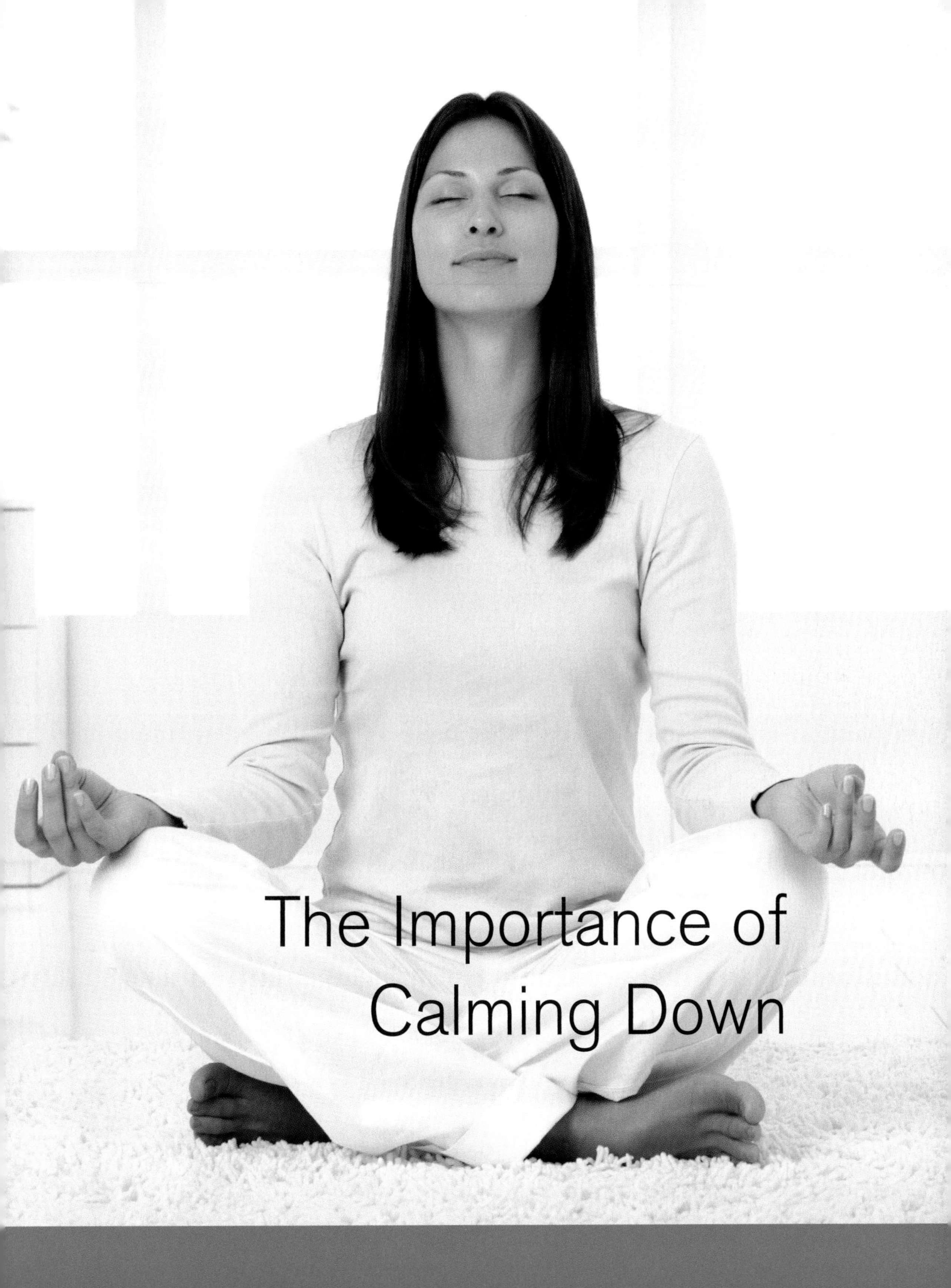

The Importance of Calming Down

CHAPTER 6

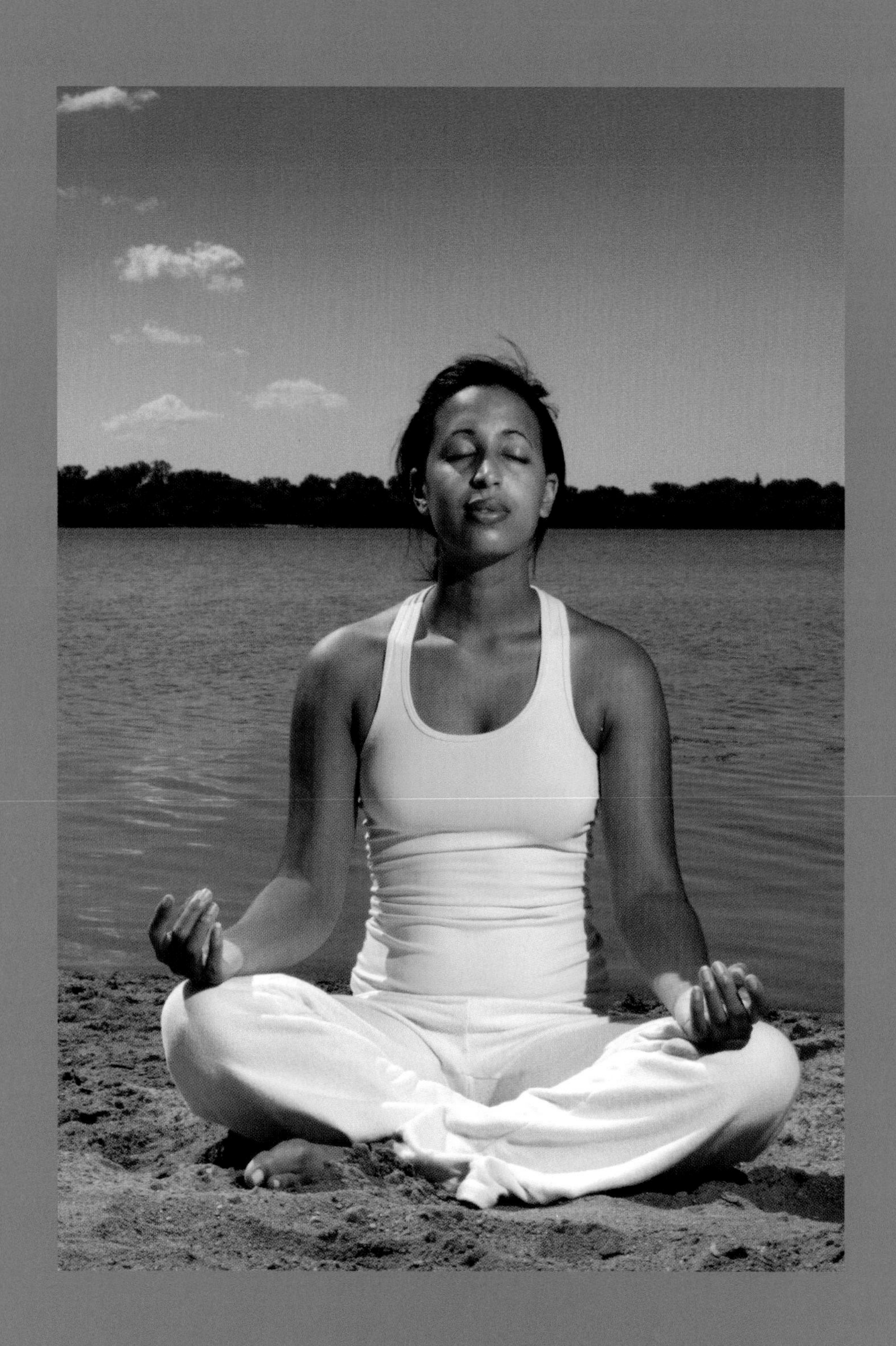

Calming Down

While the physical body is an intricate and holistic system, to really understand beauty in-depth we must examine our emotional being. Our self-awareness increases as we realize the immediacy with which our emotions affect our bodies and our skin. Both modern medicine and holistic practices agree that stress is detrimental to our health. It is surprising how beneficial it is to simply *Calm Down.*

How Damaging is Emotional Stress?

Chronic stress lowers the whole immune system. In today's pressure-ridden culture, the majority of a physician's appointments are said to be due to stress-related illnesses. How does stress deplete us, and how does this relate to holistic beauty?

There is a glow to healthy individuals that naturally draws us to them. Being well-rested is a vital part of that radiance. Stress-related fatigue depletes our adrenals, influencing our overall demeanor and sometimes causing depression.

Adrenals and Stress

The adrenal glands are located above the kidneys, which control the holding and releasing of water. They secrete adrenaline when the body is under stress. Adrenaline protects us by providing extra energy to combat danger; however, when the adrenals are over-stimulated long-term, they cause the kidneys to also be over-stimulated and lose water. Our body's response to this is to hoard water in order to prevent depletion. This creates heaviness in the body along with puffiness of the eyes and face. Often people mistake this water-retention for weight gain. Edema is a Kapha imbalance: the holding of water.

Some health practitioners believe the adrenals are so important that we must treat them before any other healing can occur. Because they regulate our stress and energy levels, improving their function helps all of our other organs.

Stress and Skin Dehydration

One of the most common causes of dehydrated skin is the stress of an overactive mind. As mentioned previously, our adrenal function directly relates to our body's water-regulation. While this can take the form of water-retention, this water-retention is created by long-term water-loss. Because our bodies are accustomed to losing water, we begin to store excess fluid to compensate. But this fluid is not distributed as usual and does not nourish our tissues.

Effects of dehydration:

- Premature aging
- Oil imbalance and acne
- Fine lines
- Poor product absorption
- Dry, flaky, chapped skin
- Sensitivity
- Aggravation of rosacea and eczema
- Accentuates hyper-pigmentation
- Reactive skin
- Dullness of complexion
- Clogged pores

Stress also can contribute to constipation as it causes tension in the intestinal muscles. As we know, constipation is dehydrating. Excess stress leads to Vata aggravation which displays itself through dehydration, weight loss and memory loss. This can also lead to the dysfunction of other doshas (ex. Kapha water retention, Pitta inflammation).

We can diagnose stress-related dehydration easily as it is not easily curable through applying creams or drinking liquids. For this reason facials are dually beneficial; not only can they treat the skin, but also impart relaxation.

Stress and Redness

Type A personalities often exhibit excess redness. Repression of anger and other stresses create unreleased internal heat which increases the heart rate and dilates the capillaries. Burst and broken capillaries are more of a cardiovascular disorder than a skin condition. Blushing when we are embarrassed, or flushing when exercising, are forms of acute stress that translate into inflammation.

Stress and Hormonal Imbalance

The body is a holistic system – this a statement echoed throughout this book, and the hormonal system reinforces this. When we are under stress, adrenaline is produced as a priority, and the constant need for it neglects the production of other hormones which throws our whole system out of balance. This can cause underproduction of progesterone, affecting menstruation and fertility. Stress can also contribute to hormone-related acne due to excess testosterone which it also encourages production

Stress and Fat

When we are under stress we crave calories, especially from sugar. According to Ayurveda, this is related to a Pitta imbalance, often connected to the heart. Ambitious, perfectionist high-Pitta people crave sweets because they taste cool in contrast to their heat.

An overactive mind stresses the body and creates a desire for calories, adding to our society's current problem with obesity. This is why kids who spend a lot of time on computers are often addicted to chocolate bars: sugar satiates the brain.

Stress also causes weight gain due to cortisol which the adrenals produce as well as adrenaline. Cortisol can also cause weight gain around the stomach area, creating a fat tire in the mid-section.

Note: Coritisol is an anti-inflammatory intended to aid trauma and to soothe inflammation in stressful situations. Dermatologists often prescribe hydrocortisone cream to heal skin reactions including rosacea. As previously mentioned, these creams are harmful long-term, making us dependent on external cortisone and compromising our immune response.

Stress and Regeneration

Overproduction of adrenaline provides an unnatural source of energy. This often results in insomnia, producing an unwelcome "second wind" even when we are exhausted. Without ample sleep, the body finds it difficult to regenerate our skin and tissues. In these situations, whatever energy exists goes into maintenance, and when all reserves are used, we crash, often resulting in disease.

Stress and Emotional Well-being

A commitment to relaxation is a commitment to self-respect and self-love. We often neglect this in order to tend to our families and our careers. We even feel guilty when we make ourselves a priority. Being a martyr does not do anyone any good and can cause long-term depletion.

It is important to make time to unwind and reduce stress. Remember, we are not only our most beautiful when we are at peace, but we are also in the most positive state to be the best parents, spouses and team members.

When discussing stress reduction, I always remember a treatment I performed on a very composed middle aged woman – her very first facial. After I cleansed her skin, we had a nice chat about its condition. She told me she needed a simple regime because she was the mother of three boys, leaving her hardly any time to cleanse her face morning and night.

During the portion of the facial in which I do an extensive neck and shoulder massage, she started to weep. "I don't remember the last time I was this relaxed," she said. Though I didn't know if her tears were of joy or of sadness over her self-neglect, releasing her emotions through her body marked a change in the way she would live her life.

Whatever is taxing us, we need to make ourselves a priority. Long-term stress sacrifices our health, our ability to perform, our happiness and, therefore, our appearance.

Stress Reduction

Some ways to reduce stress are:

- Regular exercise
- Time spent in nature/ outdoors
- Meditation
- Regular meals
- Body massage and other relaxing treatments

Personally, I also find engaging in arts and culture nourishing for my soul. By taking my mind away from the trivial and the concerns of the ego, it reminds me of the powerful beauty of creative expression.

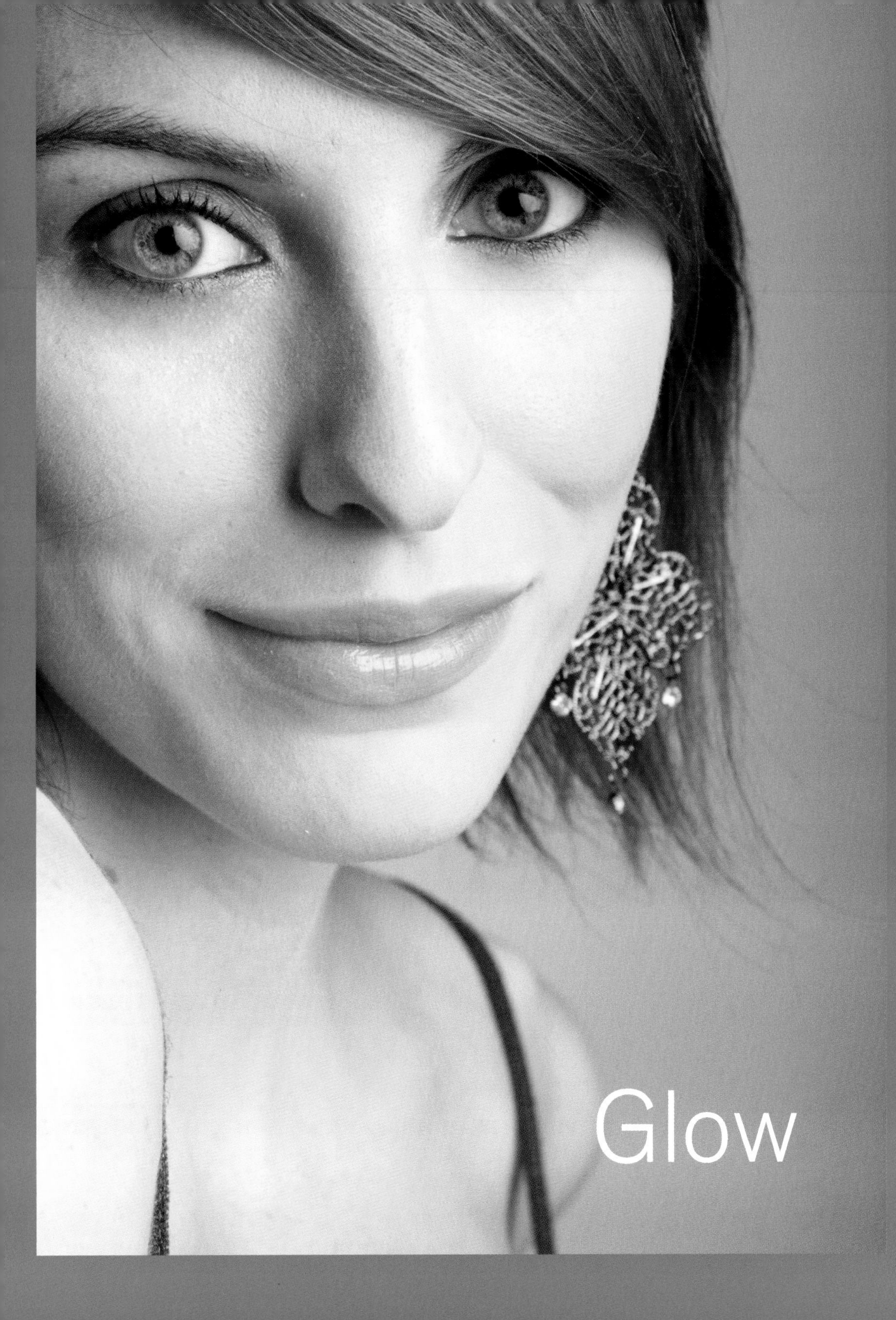

Glow

CHAPTER 7

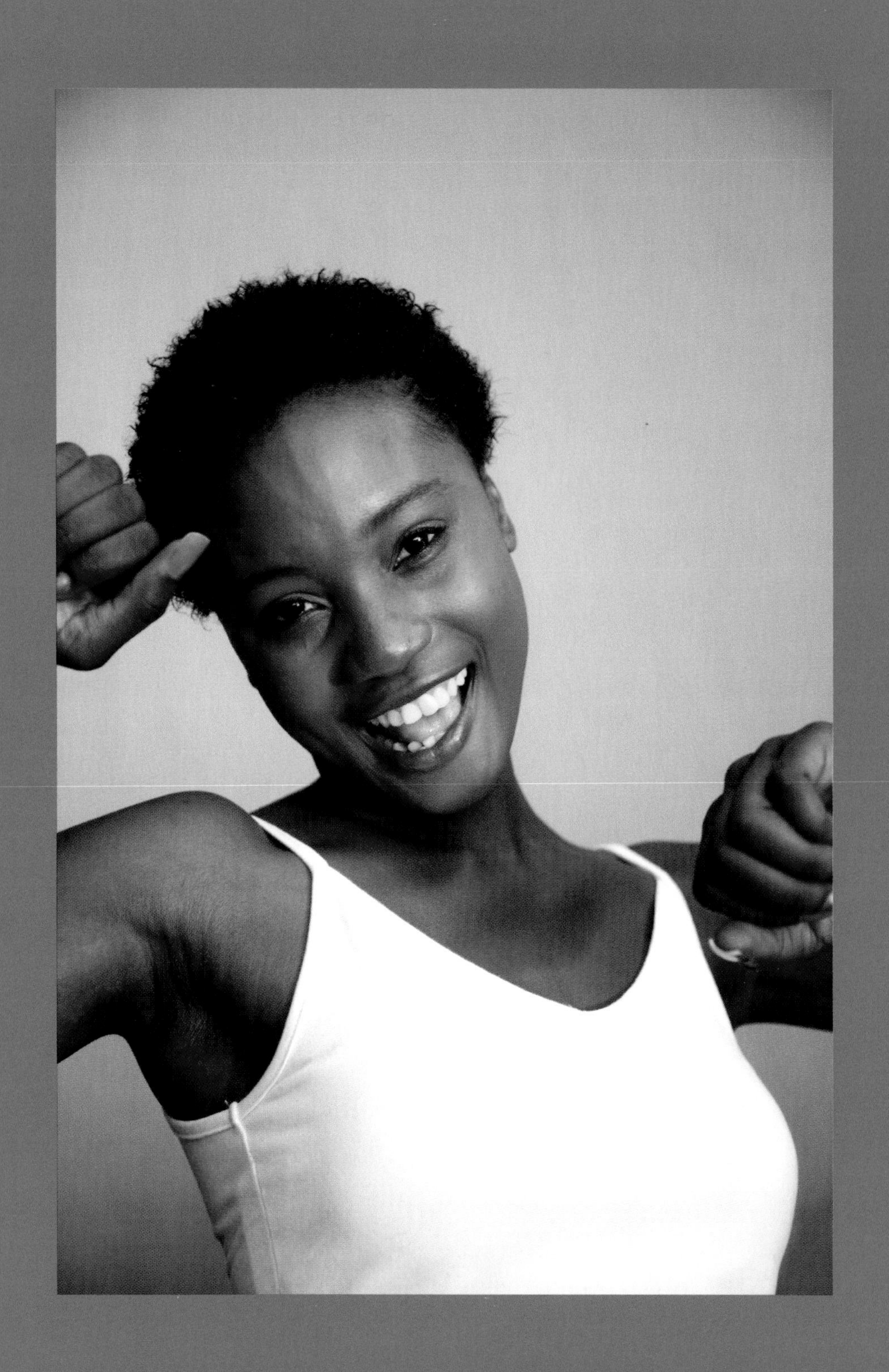

Golden Rules for that Golden Glow

Now that you understand what our skin reveals about us, and how it is affected by the health of our body, mind and emotions, we can concentrate on how to keep it beautiful through a long-term, holistic perspective.

The following is a guide to healthy and beautiful skin, using modern science in synergy with Eastern medicine.

Master the Balancing Act of Oil vs. Water

How do we balance our skin? What does "balance" mean?

We need to start with the right mindset. Instead of focusing on things we dislike and want to eliminate, such as acne and wrinkles, we should visualize what we want – *glowing, healthy skin*. From this perspective we can gently balance and heal.

What is Preventing our Skin from Being Healthy?

Our skin is constantly striving to be "normal." In the most basic terms, this means achieving a healthy balance of oil and water, allowing it to be a barrier, absorber, eliminator and regenerator. When we know which (or both) we lack, it is easy to make skincare decisions to correct this imbalance.

Just to clarify, we are going to be talking about natural vegetable oils (organic, unprocessed ones are even better) and water (preferably plant-waters). Chemically-based systems will only further imbalance the skin because of their stripping and congesting properties.

Skin health is basically a balancing act between the water it contains and the protective oil shielding and lubricating its surface.

When diagnosing the skin, it is beneficial to overlook the traditional categories of dry, oily and combination. Many people with oil on their skins' surfaces are actually dry-skinned with a self-induced oil over-production. The opposite can also happen. Some people attempt to treat dryness by slathering on oil-rich products when they really suffer from dehydration: a lack of water.

Oily Dehydrated

This skin type lacks water making it feel tight, yet greasy. Sometimes it even flakes while there is oil on its surface. It is prone to pore-congestion because its oil dries and hardens due to the underlying lack of water. A common misconception is that oily skins should never be moisturized; when in fact, they need hydration to prevent them from over-producing. Therefore, dehydration can be the real cause of acne.

During a facial, extractions are difficult if the skin is dehydrated. In this case, the client needs to follow a hydrating regime for at least two weeks before returning for a successful pore-cleansing.

Daily Routine Essentials

1. A milk cleanser. This is ideal because astringents encourage oil-production. Martina Gebhardt's Sage Milk Cleanser is excellent since sage is purifying. If a gel cleanser is preferred, it must be gentle.
2. An alcohol-free toner such as Pure + Simple's Organic Witch Hazel Hydrosol. This will purify the skin without drying it.
3. A serum for extra water. Pure + Simple's Algae Serum is excellent because algae is especially good at holding water.
4. A medium-weight moisturizer to slow down dehydration and soften the skin's surface.

Oily Hydrated

This is the truly oily skin type (balanced Kapha). It still needs protection and moisture to maintain its beauty, so do not fall into the misconception that this skin type needs to be dried out. Any comedones (blackheads, whiteheads) can easily be extracted. This skin ages well.

Daily Routine Essentials

1. A detoxifying mask once or twice a week to draw out impurities. Dr. Hauschka has an excellent Cleansing Clay Mask which comes in powder-form. I like this because it stays fresh for a long time and can be mixed easily with a wet, hydrating mask for balance.
2. A very light moisturizer is ideal. Serums can be sufficient to maintain moisture during warm, humid months.

Dry Dehydrated

As this skin type is depleted, it needs both oil and water . This oil-dry skin type (Vata) also experiences hydration being lost too fast through evaporation and/or aging (loss of collagen). Comedones, if any, are tiny and difficult to extract.

Daily Routine Essentials

1. An anti-aging serum. Even younger skins in this category need this prevention. Pure + Simple's own Collagen Elastin Plus Serum is fabulous for moisture and anti-aging.
2. A rich, nourishing cream. We must nourish, nourish, nourish. The cream will also seal in the water from the serum. Bio-dynamic German line, Just Pure, has a Calendula Royal Jelly Cream which is Pure + Simple's most popular cream for dry, dehydrated skin.

Dry Hydrated

This skin, which is genetically oil-dry, usually occurs in younger people. It has small pores and looks thin but is actually healthy and plump with water. Because its surface is dry, it needs oil.

Daily Routine Essentials

1. An oil-rich cream or face oil to lubricate the skin's surface and serve as a protective barrier.

Combination Hydrated

This skin type is generally healthy, perhaps with excess oil in the T-zone. The flexibility of a serum and a cream should be employed. Also, regular facials are recommended to clear the pores of the T-zone without over-peeling or drying the skin.

Combination Dehydrated

This skin is oily in the T-zone, but dry in other areas of the face. It is easily congested, again this is because of a lack of water. Mixing and/or layering is important for this skin type.

Daily Routine Essentials

1. Lavender for balancing oil-production. An organic lavender hydrosol is recommended as a toner.
2. A serum and a medium-weight cream can be mixed or applied each to a specific area depending on need.

Normal Skin

Perfectly normal skin simply needs gentle maintenance to prevent future imbalances.

Using a natural skincare regime is important to prevent inducing other skin conditions.

Daily Routine Essentials

1. Gentle and neutral cleansers and toners (neutral means medium-weight and not treatment-based). Never use bar soap. This is an across-the-board rule easily ignored when you have normal skin.
2. A simple, neutral moisturizer.

Hydration:
The First Line of Defense

We have discussed the balance of oil and water, but now will further examine the role of water in skin health. Like every plant and being on this Earth, we need hydration, both on our skin's surface and inside our bodies to function properly.

Definition: Dehydration is the lack of water.
Dry skin is lacking in oil.

Effects of Dehydration

Fine Lines

We all know that lack of water causes fine lines – superficial dehydration. These are not laugh lines or deep wrinkles (caused by the breakdown or loss of collagen and elastin) and are easily minimized with hydration.

Acne

People rarely think of dehydration as a cause of acne; therefore, they typically treat this condition with drying agents or so-called "oil-free" products. Not only does this deplete and weaken the skin, leaving it vulnerable to acne infection, but it also inhibits the skin's own oil flow.

Because of extreme dehydration, secreted oil hardens on the skin's surface, resulting in clogged pores. This encourages the skin to produce more oil.

Sensitivity

Sensitivity is worsened by dehydration, which is why I advocate heavy moisturizing for a few days before waxing or the use of hydrating, and gentle exfoliating treatments. I also recommend steaming thoroughly before pore-extraction in order to minimize redness.

Skin redness, from dilated and broken capillaries, is more common in dehydrated skin. Think of how tight the skin feels when lacking moisture. Broken capillaries become brittle and break in these environments. Compare them to the way a dry elastic band breaks when expanded but will be supple and flexible when moist.

Absorption

Dehydrated skin not only lacks water, but also finds it difficult to absorb moisture. This makes many of my clients think their cream or lotion is too heavy.

Compare the skin to the Earth's soil. Ground which is hard and dry will not absorb water as successfully as soil which is moist. That is because the dryness creates a crust-like barrier. It is the same with the skin. So, take a deep breath and keep using a super-hydrating moisturizer. Exfoliation will also help as it will enable moisture to penetrate more deeply.

Extracting Clogged Pores

When skin is dehydrated, it not only clogs more easily, but extractions will be more difficult because dry skin holds onto its congestion. This is explained through another Earth analogy. Weeds in moist earth are much easier to pull than those in dry soil; dry soil hangs onto the weeds, even breaking them at the stem and leaving the root. Using extra steam before the extractions will help. This can also be applied when waxing hair from dehydrated skin. To ensure removal of the hair's root, exfoliate and hydrate the skin a day before waxing.

Ailments

Specific skin ailments like eczema, rosacea, psoriasis and dermatitis are aggravated by dehydration. Sometimes eczema is triggered when oil is applied to extremely dehydrated skin. This is because water is needed, not oil which increases heat (inflammation/Pitta).

Allergic reactions and chapped skin from chaffing can also be triggered or intensified by dehydration. This is due to the skin's immunity being low, as well as to the sensitivity and dehydration discussed above. The skin cannot heal if it does not have water. With the exception of fungus, most of its ailments need nourishment for rebuilding and regenerating.

How to hydrate

Topical hydration provides the most immediate fix. The right combination of water-based and oil-based products is so important. If the skin is not being hydrated, or if you are using chemicals, it is nearly impossible for the skin to maintain moisture. This means using natural products without petroleum and sodium laurel sulfate must be part of any replenishing program. If the skin is still dehydrated while using nourishing skincare, other factors must be examined.

Internal measures

The most obvious way to hydrate is by drinking water, yet some of us drink plenty of water and are still dehydrated. As one of my clients joked, "I could drown in all I drink in a day, yet my skin is still dehydrated!" Ayurveda describes this condition as Vata excess. Eating hydrating food is beneficial – soups, stews, vegetables with cellular fiber and high water content. This should be combined with avoiding dehydrating liquids, such as coffee and alcohol, and dehydrating foods such as starch and meat.

Taking oils and fats is another way of helping hydration. Oils hold water, as well as lubricate the intestines, making it easier to eliminate. A clean system is important for hydration.

Pittas can dehydrate despite high water-consumption because internal heat dries water up. Dehydrated Pittas often feel heat and dryness in the mouth and throat. Drinking liquid which tastes slightly sweet (from fruit, vegetables, complex carbohydrates, but not white refined sugar) can serve as a Pitta coolant, as can drinking water charged with fruit and vegetable essences. Some people soak healing crystals in drinking water to "charge" it with healing energy while others find that our own "energetic intentions" effectively charge the water. Note: Pittas have difficulty digesting oils.

Decrease Stress

As previously discussed, stress is dehydrating. Spa treatments can be helpful, but lifestyle and mindset changes are the long-term solution to this kind of dehydration.

Circulation

Poor blood flow deprives skin cells of nourishment. Our extremities are most affected because they are furthest from the heart, resulting in dry hands, cracked heels, and flaky scalp. Poor circulation and dehydration cause an accumulation of toxins that create cellulite. Improved circulation can be achieved through exercise and massage.

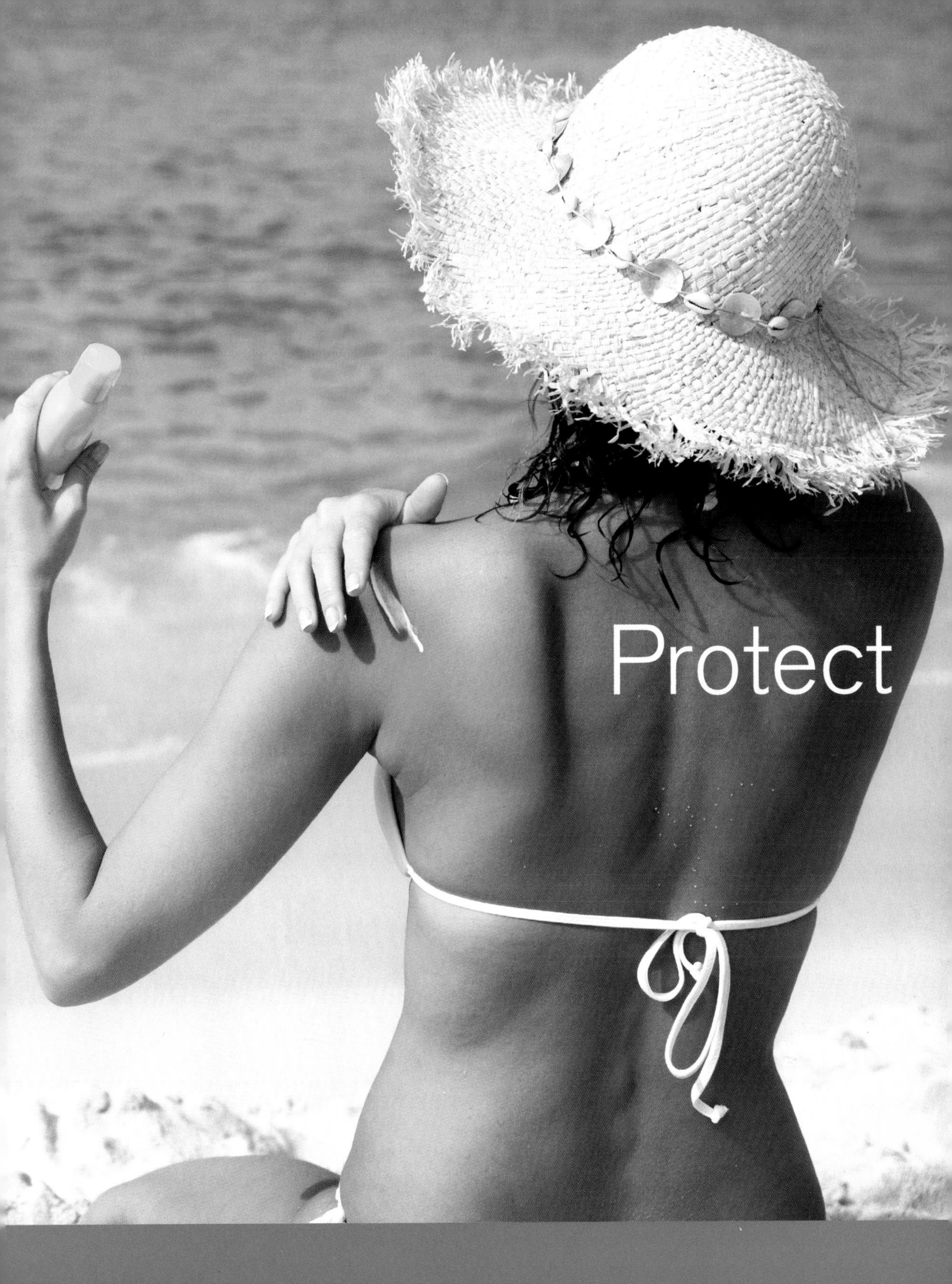

Protect

CHAPTER 8

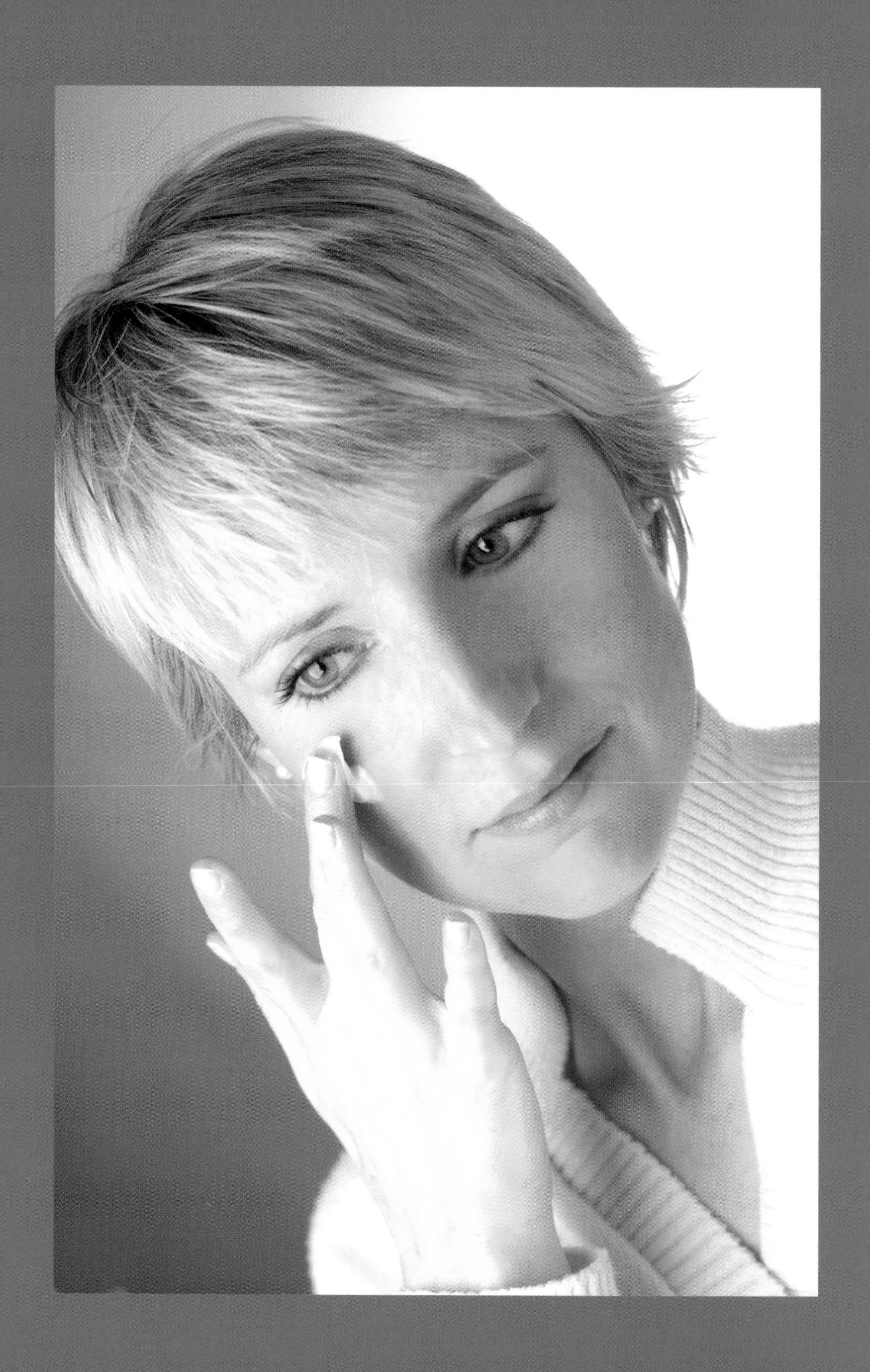

Protect Yourself!

After hydrating, good oil-protection is key. Even the healthiest skin needs protection. Requirements differ with genetics, geography and exposure. Wind, cold, heat, dryness, sun, dirt, indoor climate-control and manmade pollution all assault healthy skin, requiring balancing measures to restore and maintain beauty.

Four Protectors for our Skin

1. A good **Moisturizer** for our skin-type, to guard against environmental conditions and dehydration.
2. **Sunscreen** or Sun Protection Factor Products (SPF). This is for free radical and skin cancer prevention. Some nut-oils have a natural SPF.
3. A **Serum** to keep cells plump so skin can act as a barrier against bacteria and dirt.
4. A gentle **Cleanser** to cleanse away dirt and pollution (pollution and exhaust fumes can cause skin damage). This also will not strip our skin's defenses for that "squeaky-clean feeling."

Skin Protection and Healing

Our skin needs protection to shield it from damage and depletion. Studies have also proven that if the skin is protected from trauma, it has the ability to rebuild and regenerate itself even without rejuvenating or anti-aging treatments, though they are still beneficial.

Moisturizer as a Shield

Moisturizing our skin is not only important for hydration but also for protection. The more oil-based the moisturizer, the more it acts as a barrier between the skin and the elements. It also becomes a seal, locking in moisture and preventing water from evaporating through the pores as sweat.

Cleansing Away the Damage

We also protect our skin by avoiding harsh chemicals and toxic pollutants. People often ask me if they need to wash their faces twice a day. The answer is a definite "Yes!" When clients are reluctant to do so, I insist on cleansing at least at night. We do not want the day's pollution and dirt sitting in our pores overnight. As well as clogging, they trigger breakouts, cause inflammation and are absorbed into our bodies.

External Environment

As the seasons change, so do the requirements of our skin. More protection is needed in winter, which is why we should change to richer creams. In summer, a lighter lotion can be used, but protection from dehydration is essential. Summer-time protection shifts focus from dehydration to guarding against UV damage.

Sun Protection

Sunscreen is probably our best-known skin protection. The sun has been cited as the primary source of hyper-pigmentation, aging and, of course, skin cancer. While the need for a sun block is indisputable, we must make the right choices when selecting one.

While humans require fifteen minutes of sun a day to obtain adequate Vitamin D for healthy bones and teeth, longer exposure can damage the skin's cells, causing premature aging. This occurs when the sun's rays penetrate into the inner skin layers, damaging collagen and elastin fibers. As a result, sunscreens are a new essential for proactive beauty. Fortunately, they have not been shown to impede Vitamin D absorption.

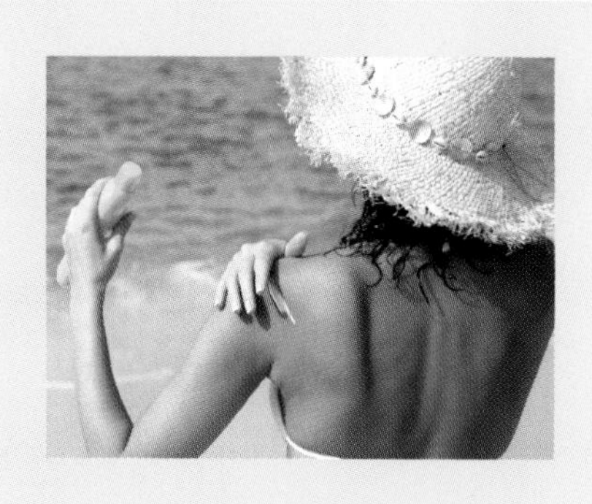

Sunblocks are available in the form of lotions, sprays and mineral makeup.

Chemical Sunscreens vs. Natural Sun Blocks

Sunscreens are of two types: natural blocks, using zinc and titanium, which create a physical barrier against UV rays, and chemical ones which neutralize and absorb UV rays into the skin's tissues. While chemical sunblocks are popular because they are easier to formulate into bases and cosmetics, natural sunscreens are generally less toxic, less irritating and cause fewer allergies.

Safety Concerns

The highest SPF in most natural sun blocks is SPF 30. While we, in our sun-fearing society, may wish to increase that number, high level chemical sunscreens can actually heighten the likelihood of cancer because they contain proven carcinogens.

Many sunscreen agents, like octyl-methoxycinnamate, octyl-dimethyl-PABA (OD-PABA), benzophenone-3, homosalate (HMS) and 4-Methyl-benzylidene camphor (4-MBC) are also endocrine disrupters, upsetting the body's hormone balance. In particular, they have been shown to disrupt levels of estrogen, even allowing traces of their chemicals into breast milk. The higher the SPF, the more toxic, which is why there is movement to outlaw any higher than 30. This is already the case in Australia.

Natural sunscreens sit on the skin's surface like a shield. This means they do not need to be reapplied to stay effective. Chemical sunscreens need reapplication every one to two hours as the sunscreen agents they contain become inactive. Researchers have found that people who are unaware of this get more sun damage because they are under the illusion they are protected.

Studies have also found that people who wear sunscreen have a higher incidence of skin cancer because they spend more time in the sun under the belief that reapplication restarts the protecting action; however, once erythema (redness from burning) begins, reapplication does not stop it. You must reapply the block *before* this happens and take breaks from the sun, letting your skin cool. Remember, with each reapplication, more chemicals are absorbed.

Other Benefits of Natural Sun Blocks

Natural sun blocks, using zinc and titanium minerals, provide a beauty benefit as well as one for health. Zinc possesses soothing, disinfecting properties. This means it is anti-inflammatory for sensitive skin and anti-bacterial for acne. Many chemical sunscreens clog pores and irritate due to their toxic and petroleum content.

Understanding What is Important: Measuring Sun Protection

The general misconception is that the higher the SPF the more protection, but SPF only describes how long the sunscreen will remain active. It is the amount of time it takes for skin to burn, multiplied by the SPF protection number. Example: if it takes five minutes to burn without sunscreen, with an SPF 15 it will take 75 minutes (15 x 5 minutes).

Many people also assume that the higher SPF provides more protection. Actually, the difference in filtration of UV rays between SPF 15 and SPF 30 is minute – 96 per cent compared to 98 per cent.

As mentioned, sun-conscious countries like Australia have banned sunscreens over SPF 30.

The high concentration of chemicals also cause free radicals.

UVA table:

Ray Type	Over-exposure Effects
UVA	• (longest rays) • Damage to skin, • Premature Aging, • Skin Cancer
UVB	• Eurythmea (Redness from Burning)
UVC	• Skin Cancer

Be Gentle

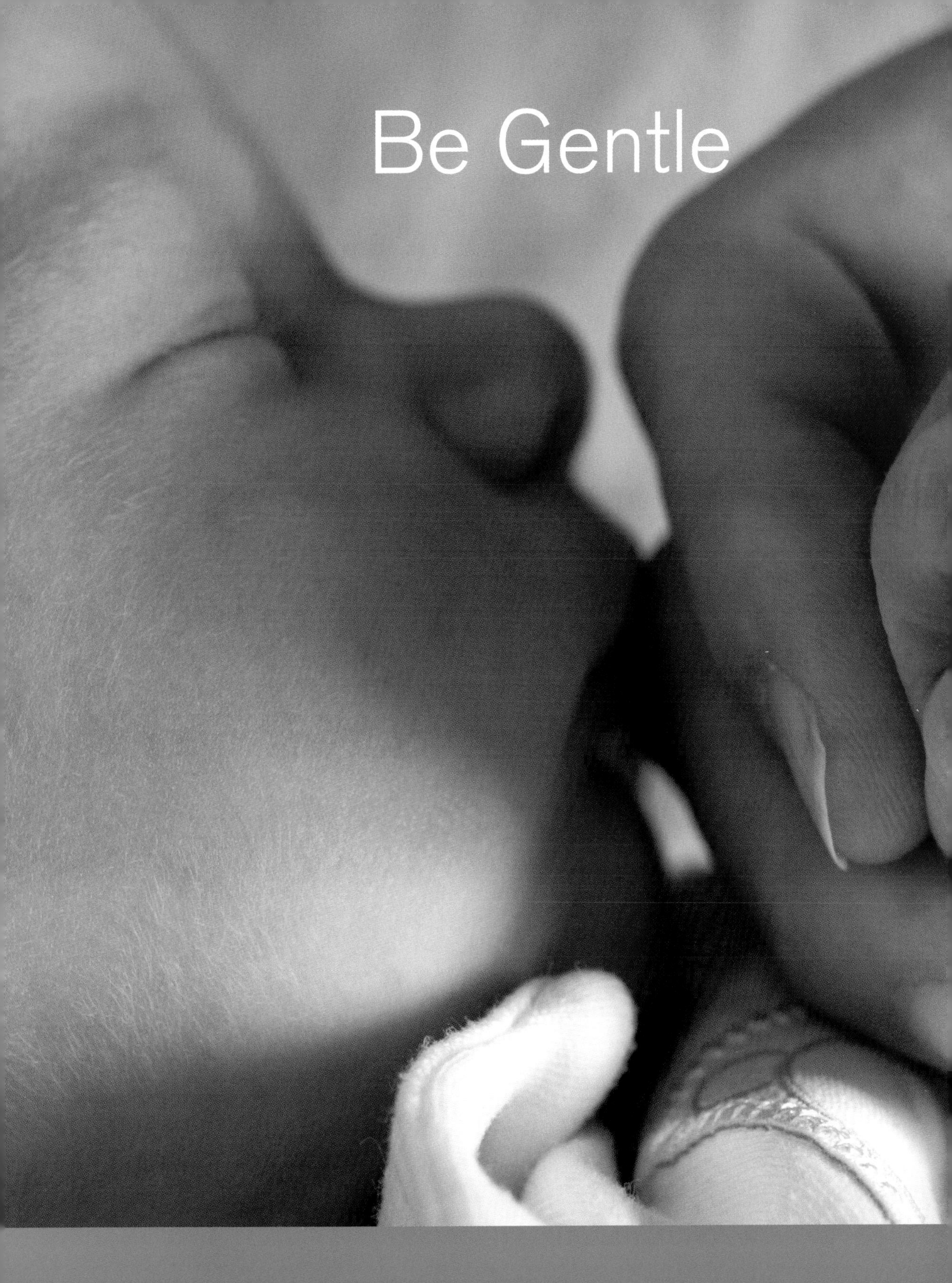

CHAPTER 9

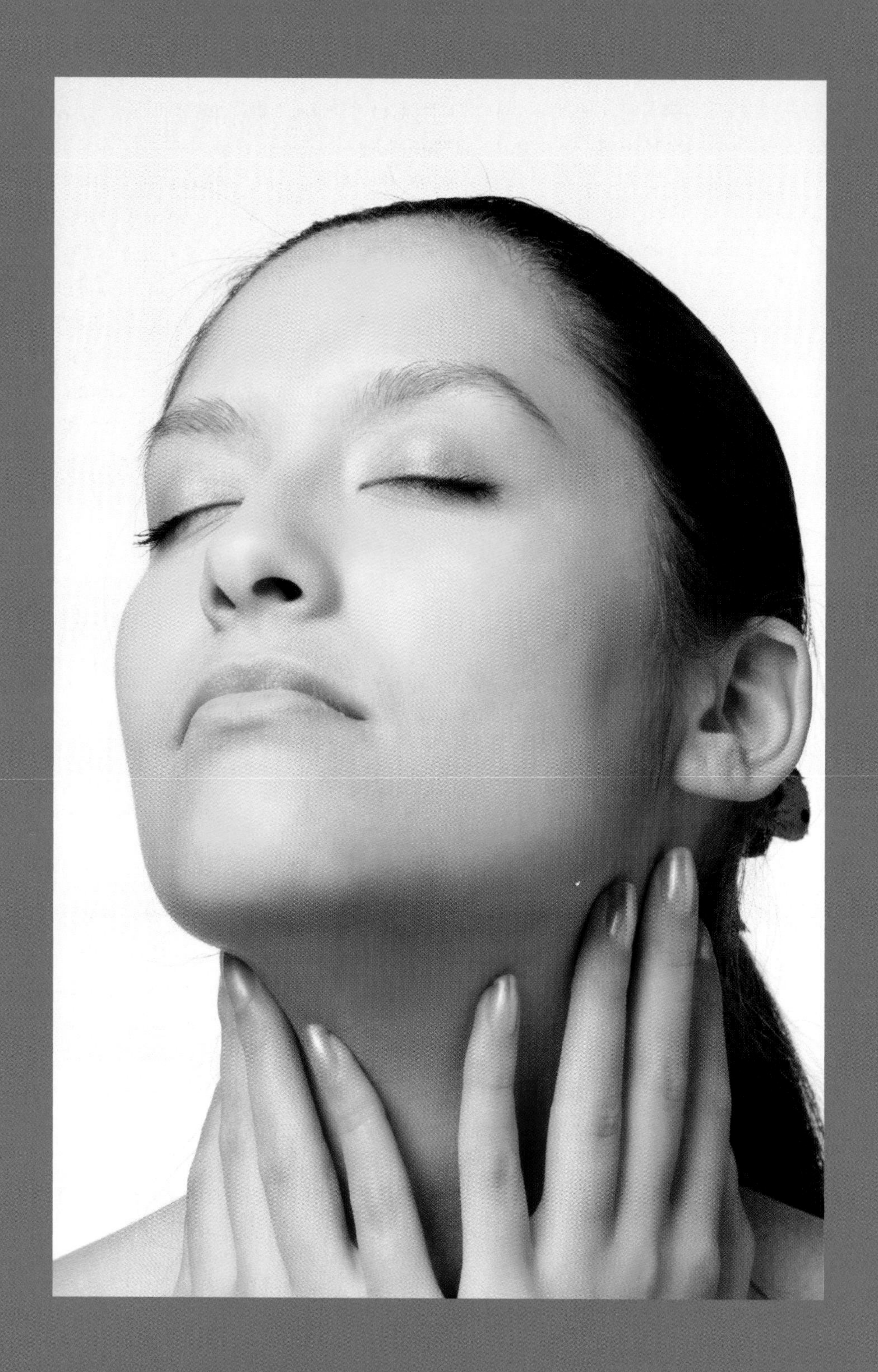

Be Gentle

We must think of our skin as a gatekeeper to our internal organs. It is extremely delicate, so being gentle is very important.

We live in a culture which encourages us to be tough on ourselves as a method of getting results. I believe this not only affects our self-esteem, but crosses over into our grooming habits. We often want to over-wash, over-scrub and over-dry our skin to rid ourselves of dirt, blemishes and the like. North Americans especially love to over-exfoliate, creating oil imbalances, dehydration, sensitivities and irritation.

Stripping the skin disrupts its acid mantle – the coating of sebum on its surface, made up of fatty acids and alcohol, waxes, salts and lactic acid. Since this mantle creates a barrier against bacteria, over-washing decreases the skin's resilience, immunity and general health. Even for acne, I prescribe a gentle regime because stripping the skin provokes the production of excess oil.

Pampering Principles for the Skin

1. **Avoid chemical ingredients:** Chemical dyes, perfumes and detergents aggravate and damage the skin. Especially avoid sodium laurel sulfate which is so stripping that it is often used to degrease heavy machinery. Also remember, clogged and dehydrated skin is more sensitive.
2. **Avoid irritants:** Do not use products which over-stimulate or irritate. Avoid allergens. The more we stress our skin, the less healthy it becomes just as eating foods to which we have sensitivities taxes our immune systems.
3. **Avoid drying ingredients:** Even natural ingredients can be astringent. Only use drying hydrosols, essential oils and herbs when necessary. For example, using pure tea tree daily on our skin is too harsh, unless we are trying to kill an acute infection. We must opt for something gentler like lavender as a daily antiseptic. For ultra-sensitive skin, also avoid pure peppermint or rosemary. It is better to use essences which are heavily diluted or hydrolats.
4. **Stop over-exfoliating and over-washing:** This leaves the acid mantle depleted and abused. Also, use a product which respects the delicacy of the skin.

10 Soothing Ingredients

- German Chamomile
- Sandalwood
- Organic Coconut Oil
- Calendula
- Melissa
- Cornflower
- Rose
- Aloe Vera
- Oat beta glucan
- Zinc oxide

Gentle Touch

Even when touching your skin, be gentle – love it. Do not rub it abrasively. When undergoing extractions, make sure your esthetician is also gentle. Comedones should never be forced out. Only extract those which leave the pores easily.

Choosing gentle treatments and products, as well as using a gentle touch in our daily skin-care, does much to maintain our youthfulness.

Our Delicate Areas: Eyes, Lips and Neck

Be especially careful with the skin of the eyes, lips and neck due to their more delicate nature. The tissue in these areas are often thinner and more easily damaged.

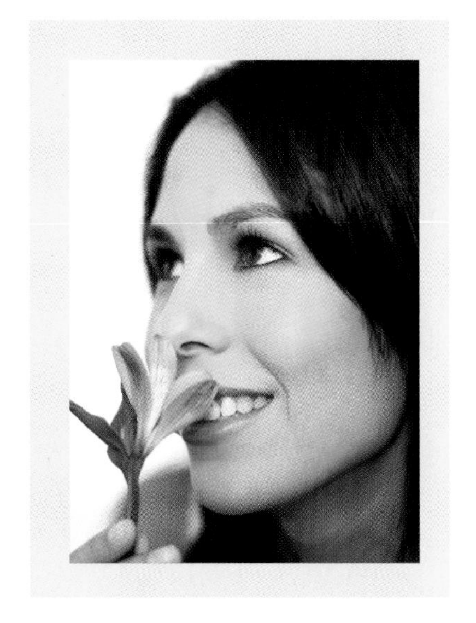

Eyes: the Window to the Soul

Our eyes are one of the first things others notice about us, and usually the first area to show aging. Many of us have very sensitive eyes due to genetics, eye strain or poor daily care. The success of expensive creams in tiny jars demonstrates how much we treasure beautiful eyes.

Sensitive Eyes

The eyes are the domain of Pitta, which governs heat, redness, irritation and inflammation. Sensitive eyes are often due to excess Pitta, causing dryness and burning. A cooling, hydrating eye cream is an excellent aid, but many people have reactions to these products. Sometimes eye-stinging can be mistaken for a reaction when it is just an initial response to the product's cooling properties. If stinging quickly dissipates, the eyes are simply adjusting to the anti-inflammatory action. Cool compresses will also reduce heat in the eyes.

Also, for those with sensitive eyes, less is more where makeup is concerned. Pure ingredients and natural colors are a big help as they do not have irritating dyes. Organic Kajals from the German company Lakshmi Ayurvedic Beauty offer an effective solution to reactive eyes. The black color comes from the carbon of burnt organic ghee (clarified butter) which is an excellent anti-inflammatory.

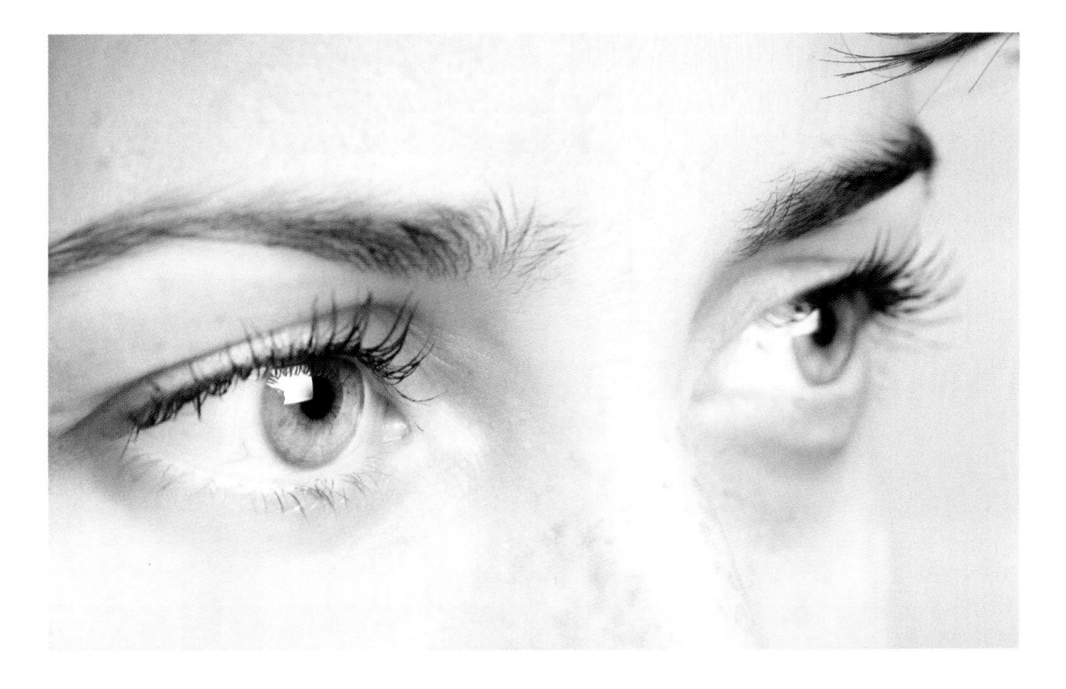

Dark Circles

There are many causes for "raccoon eyes," but most people assume it is a genetic trait, having experienced dark circles for as long as they could remember. But while under-eye circles may be inherited, genetics may have more to do with our kidneys than our eye areas.

While the lower lip of the lower lid is an adrenal area, the lower lid where the eye socket begins is a kidney area (feel the bone underneath your eye – this section is kidney-related). As we get older, the skin around our eyes gets saggier and baggier with dark circles becoming more pronounced. This is because the kidneys are Vata organs, and the Vata dosha is much stronger as we enter old age. Those of use with high Vata often have eye circles from even a young age.

Another cause of dark circles is deoxygenated blood. Blood without oxygen is dark causing bluishness under the eyes. Using products with antioxidants can be very effective as well as using an eye cream that promotes circulation. Arnica, along with other stimulating plants, is excellent. This also aids lymphatic drainage and moves stagnant blood which are other causes of under-eye circles.

Puffy Eyes

Puffiness is a Kapha trait. Any glandular, sinus congestion or other fluid-retention is governed by the water element. TCM dictates that water flows in a downward energy (yin), usually affecting the lower body. When puffiness is in the face, it is a combination of excess water with yang energy (because heat rises). This means Kapha and Pitta elements and toxins are causing it.

When we lack sleep, our eyes also become puffy because the lower eye lid corresponds to the adrenal glands and the kidneys (one of the most important organs in TCM). Though affected by the adrenals, the kidneys are also important for filtering and absorbing water into our bodies.

The morning is when Kapha is strongest, and that is usually when our faces are more bloated. As the day wears on, the puffiness usually drains away. Pressure point massage, when washing the face, is great for accelerating this process. Press gently around the eye-socket bones in a circular pattern, then gently press and release over the other swollen sinus areas. I find that engaging in this lymph drainage every morning helps my own Kapha puffiness to subside. Exercising in the morning also moves the lymph, stimulating drainage.

Cholesterol/ Fat Deposits

Sometimes whiteheads near the eye are from pore-clogging products. Because the pores here are smaller, it is important to use a natural product that will not clog them as tiny whiteheads often result from a buildup of product. When build-up accumulates in dehydrated skin, it dries and hardens in the pores. These little bumps, fondly referred to as cholesterol or fat deposits, sit on the skin and are difficult to extract. Often they can only be removed when punctured with a needle. It is advised that only professionals do this as the delicacy of the eye area makes it easy to damage.

Sometimes these deposits are from toxins or excess fat in our internal organs. High-fat diets, or the inability of our bodies to flush out cholesterol, can cause them.

Sometimes it is a combination of clogged pores and internal problems that cause the whiteheads. The fat deposits may disappear when a client switches to a more natural, non-clogging eye cream or gel. Many people pair this with a kidney cleanse or some other type of detox.

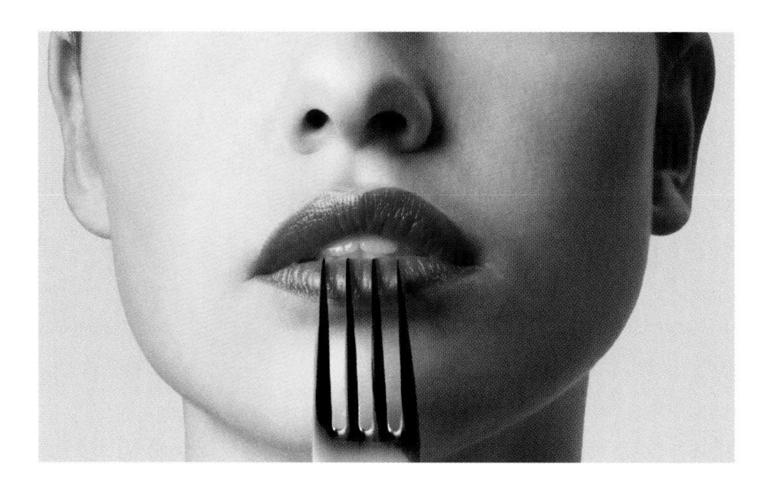

Lips: Pretty Pouts

Since the lips contain more delicate tissue than the rest of our face, they are often the first to show an allergic reaction. Because they relate to the digestive system, swelling, itchiness and irritation can indicate an internal problem. Swollen lips are a sign of extreme dehydration in the intestines and/or stomach, and display the body's attempt to retain water. (Refer back to the face-mapping section for further explanation).

While most of us see dry or flaky lips as a normal part of the winter season, they are another sign of dry internal organs. To heal them, we must hydrate internally and externally. Hydrating the gastrointestinal tract through a water-rich and easy to digest diet, as well as examining its healthiness, is important. We have already discussed the roles of the spleen, stomach and small intestine, and for further diagnosis and recommendations, it is beneficial to consult a health practitioner.

But we cannot discount the need to combat dry lips on the skin's surface. Topical protection is essential. Using mass-market lip balms with petrolatum is often counterproductive because they congest the lips' pores instead of penetrating their tissue. This is why many of us become addicted to our "chapstick." We love the sensation of moisturizing, but when that wears off, we are left with extreme dryness. Balms made of vegetable butters, waxes and oils are much more nourishing while still being protective.

Neck and Chest: the Décolletage

We often neglect the neck and décolletage (upper chest), which are early areas for showing aging. The delicate, thinner skin here is more prone to sagging, sunspots and wrinkling. While I do not think it is necessary to buy products specifically for the neck, I do recommend caring for it with serums and creams as religiously as we do our faces. I personally use my facecare regime on my décolletage.

SPF protection, with a mineral-based sun block, is especially important as this area is so vulnerable to sun exposure.

Decongest

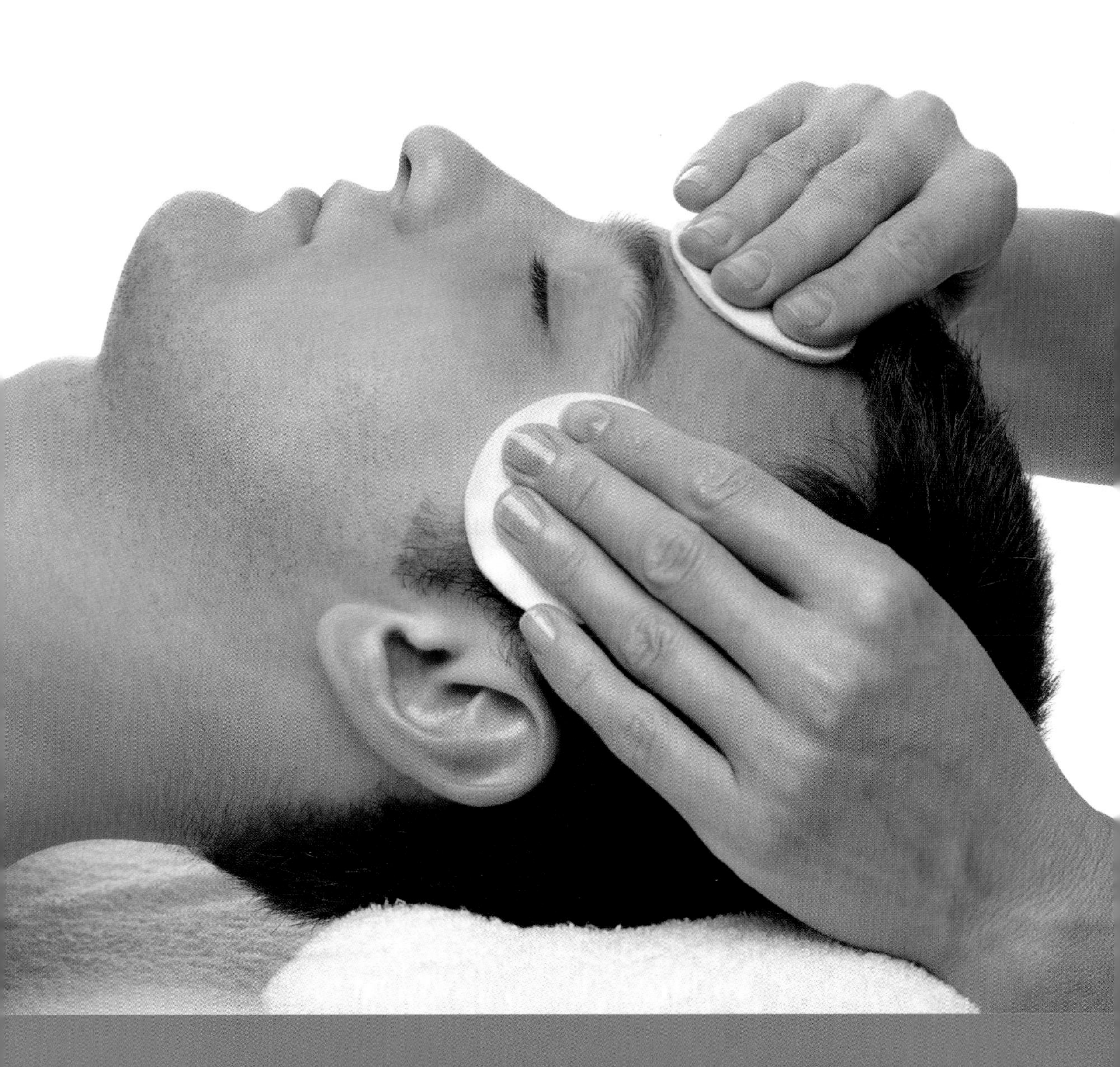

CHAPTER 10

Decongest

When the pores are clear, the skin can absorb, sebum can flow freely, detoxification is not inhibited, and a smooth texture is maintained.

If skin is hydrated and protected with healthy moisturizers, it should not become congested. When we care for our skin and it still gets congested, it is due to:

- Stress
- Changes in weather
- Our diet and digestion
- Illness
- Medication
- Genetics and our doshas

That being said, for those of us who live in urban settings with daily exposure to smog and pollution, preventing blocked pores is nearly impossible without help.

Ways to Decongest

Extraction

The quickest and most effective way to unclog pores is through extraction. Squeezing and picking should be done during a facial treatment, after the pores have been softened with hydrating serums, peels and steam or hot towels.

It is best to have extractions done by an experienced professional who will know how to extract the skin without bruising, scarring or spreading bacteria. This is especially important for those of us with sensitive or problem skin. After extractions are finished, the skin must be purified with a natural antiseptic (such as witch hazel) and the pores should be tightened with a treatment mask.

When done correctly, extractions keep the pores clean, small and fine. A monthly facial is fundamental to a healthy complexion.

Exfoliation

Exfoliation is great for preventing congestion. Removing dead skin promotes cell turnover, oxygenates the skin and improves circulation. Technological advances have produced many forms of exfoliation to fit our skin's goals and needs.

Types of Exfoliation

Manual Scrubs

Manual scrubs contain an abrasive agent to physically exfoliate our skin. Knowledge of the agent is important as some can scratch and damage our skin. The gentlest and most effective are jojoba pearls (wax beads).

Chemical Peels

Whether using AHA, BHA, glycolic acid, lactic acid or one of the newer, more intense peels, chemical exfoliants do not require manual scrubbing. Despite being called "chemical," they may utilize naturally derived acids to digest surface skin cells. At Pure + Simple, we use corn-derived lactic acid and natural fruit acids in our skin-refining products. The base of a peel is also very important as natural ingredients are gentler and penetrate more effectively.

Apply peels with caution. Frequent use makes the skin more vulnerable to UV rays, as well as causing sensitivity and irritation. This can also lead to hyper-pigmentation. The percentage level of the agent must also be carefully monitored. When I had acne, I was given 70 per cent glycolic peels performed by a dermatologist. This increased my sensitivity and damaged my skin.

All peels wound skin to promote regeneration, but with chemical peels we have less control over the depth of exfoliation and amount of irritation obtained.

Microdermabrasion

Microdermabrasion is a peeling treatment which uses a machine to buff and abrade the skin. It is referred to as a "controlled peeling" as a professional can adjust the depth of the peel by monitoring our skin throughout the treatment. A series of Microdermabrasion treatments make for an excellent anti-aging tool as they help to promote circulation, cell turnover and collagen production.

Sea-salt Microdermabrasion uses all-natural salt crystals instead of the traditionally used aluminum crystals. This is much better for our skin. Not only does the salt disinfect the skin, but it dissolves in water, unlike aluminum crystals which can leave its residue for up to two weeks.

I have extensively used both forms of Microdermabrasion. The Sea-salt Microdermabrasion gives a deeper peel with less irritation, yielding better results.

Steaming

Steaming is a fabulous, non-invasive way to sweat out congestion. As well as opening pores, it gives the skin moisture. When herbs and essential oils are added to steam, the skin absorbs them on a deeper level due to the dilation of the pores.

Steaming must be done twice per week or more to maintain results. Since it can be dehydrating, we must replenish the skin afterwards with a moisturizer/moisturizing mask. This is a great option for cystic acne skin where there is risk of spreading bacteria. Simply boil some water with the desired herbs, remove it from the heat source, then hover above it, draping a towel over your head to entrap the steam. Do this for five minutes.

Oiling and Oil Massage

Using oils to decongest the pores may seem counterintuitive, but as mentioned previously, Ayurveda recommends oils to cleanse. Ayurveda advocates ingesting large volumes of oil to cleanse the gastrointestinal (GI) tract and to draw toxins from the tissues to the organs of elimination.

Massaging with pure vegetable oils will help loosen deep-seated and embedded buildup in the skin. This ability of oil to decongest was shown to me many years ago while I was doing a facial on an acne sufferer in her late twenties who was very dehydrated yet was petrified of using moisturizer for fear of breaking out. While she had some pustules, her main problem was comedones. She was extremely clogged in her chest, her back, her shoulders and face. Because she was so dry, I decided to do an oil massage on her face, neck and shoulders, under the steam, to make the extraction easier and to prevent redness; however, as I massaged, the hardened oils in her pores began to loosen and to pop out like little corks. I had to wipe off my hands and reapply the oil multiple times. It was a remarkable experience and, needless to say, this client was not as afraid of oil after the treatment.

Prevention: The Greatest Cure

Many of us wait until we have a problem before we fix it, whether it is a major health condition, a thinning personal relationship or an issue with environmental consequences. While we may be able to heal these things, we can never reverse them to their original state. Sun damage can be faded, yet skin cells are permanently affected. Acne can be cleared, but scars can linger.

The people with the most beautiful skin are those who have been forward-thinking enough to prevent the damage. Sensitive-skinned people should take precaution against rosacea; fair-skinned people should protect against sun damage; and everyone should engage in anti-aging practices.

Furthermore, corrective treatments are not always without side-effects. Dangerous surgeries and peels can not only end up looking artificial, but they can damage cells, nerves and tissues. Pigmentation, scarring and permanent sensitivity are only some of the lasting effects of many treatments.

A preventative regime involves the combination of our other skincare principles:

- Being gentle
- Using natural skincare and cosmetics
- Protecting, hydrating, exfoliating, etc.

The Key is Awareness.

It is easy to let a problem progress through lack of monitoring. We should love and care for ourselves before emergency or trauma occurs. Listen to your body and love yourself enough to be proactive. We only receive one body and one skin each lifetime.

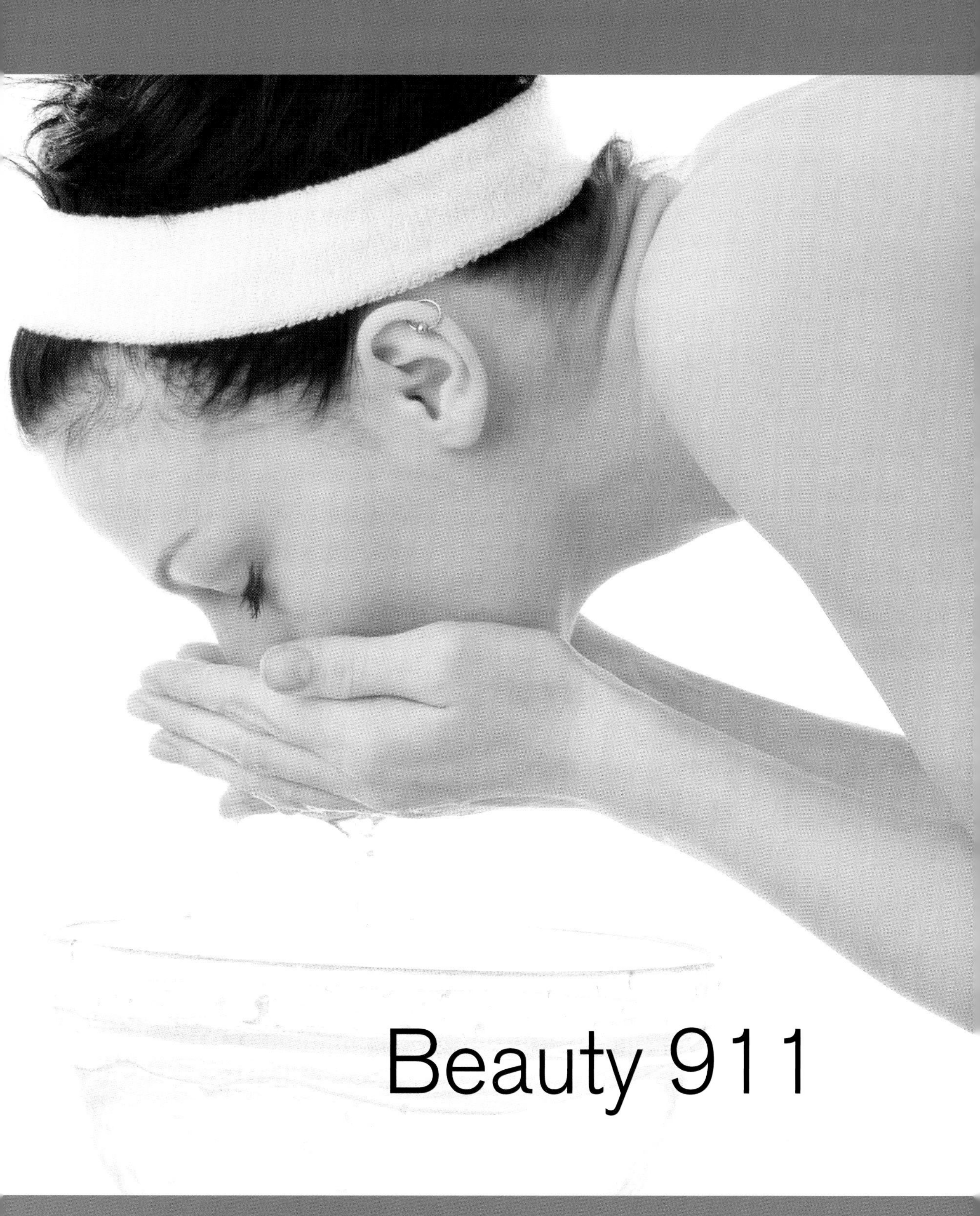

Beauty 911

CHAPTER 11

Beauty Ailments 911

Rescue your skin holistically from chronic conditions.

My passion for knowledge about skin has driven me to constantly learn. For this reason I like to stay current and to attend various seminars. During one seminar, the speaker, a "skincare authority," advised the audience of estheticians to recommend complicated and confusing regimes for their clients. This was said to ensure that we would be viewed as "experts in our field." Contrary to her advice, I feel that my usefulness relies on my ability to educate my clients. I prefer to teach them how to use easy, yet effective skincare practices to promote a more simple view of beauty. Sharing knowledge with my clients of how to identify and treat their own ailments empowers them, and that is truly good business. The following section will offer tools and education to help self-diagnose and treat the most common skin ailments.

Acne The long journey

Acne, zits, pimples, pustules, blemishes

Whatever we call them, we detest them. In this age of high stress, pollution and junk food, acne is widespread, causing even more stress. For some, it may be a minor annoyance, but for others it undermines self-image and lowers self-esteem. "I couldn't even look people in the eye," an acne client of mine once told me. Such people are prime victims for the false promise of beautiful skin from makers of "deep-pore cleansers" and "oil-free creams." I was one of those people.

The problem is that many of us are misinformed. Often acne begins in a minor way, caused by hormones, bad products or stress. It is when the frustration over breakouts starts, and we begin to squeeze and apply damaging commercial products or medications, that the problem turns into a condition.

From the beginning: What is acne?

A pimple is a clogged pore which has become infected and inflamed, turning it into a pustule. This is why the minimization of blackheads decreases acne.

Causes: Inside and Out

Clogged Pores

As explained, synthetic ingredients in skincare and makeup can clog pores. Clogging causes a comedone (black or whitehead) which is the first component of a breakout. Often acne sufferers depend on cover-up cosmetics to hide their blemishes, worsening the problem. Even when good skincare is used, the clogging effect of some commercial makeup lines prevents the skin from fully clearing.

Fear of Oil

Excess oil is the commonly blamed culprit for acne-prone skin, therefore, it is generally believed that stripping the skin of its oils will prevent and clear up blemishes. Instead, this causes dehydration, which is the root cause of overproduction of sebaceous oil, initiating a vicious cycle.

Oily skin is the most beautiful and healthiest type, if properly maintained. Its greatest need is hydration so that sebum overproduction does not solidify in the pores creating comedones.

Dehydration

Dehydration is actually the most common cause of acne. Often people break out during the seasonal change from summer into fall, or when traveling into a less-humid environment. Most people believe it is humidity that causes breakouts, but it is usually the absence of moisture.

Since we cannot control how our bodies will disperse the water we ingest, applying moisturizers is the most direct way to fight dehydration. Oil-based products will also help seal water in.

Cigarette-smoking, caffeine and alcohol are dehydrating, as well as taxing to the liver. A tip I recommend to people who like to stay out late drinking alcohol is to use a very nourishing moisturizer prior to sleep. In that way, they will minimize the consequences of skin dehydration. While sleeping early and avoiding alcohol is ideal, this boost of moisture will help compensate for bad habits.

Sun

Abundant sun exposure can cause breakouts for high Pittas because the heat pushes out toxins. The sun also stimulates the sebaceous glands, sometimes causing breakouts. Too much sun will also dehydrate the skin.

Sun burns traumatize the skin and tax its immunity, this leaves it vulnerable to more blemishes.

Toxins and Liver Overload

Chronic acne (especially adult acne) is almost always an indication of an imbalance in the liver, and even the purest skincare products cannot heal this.

The liver is also the body's filtration system. If it is overloaded, it will not absorb or filter properly, and excess toxins will spill into other areas. This translates into pimples, as the skin is the largest organ of detoxification, and toxins which cannot be filtered and eliminated will purge through it.

Sleep helps to regenerate and detoxify the liver. According to the natural rhythms of our body, the liver usually detoxifies from one to three o'clock in the morning making sleep during these hours important.

Pitta governs the liver which plays a huge role in hormone filtration. The liver also is closely related to the emotion of anger, making those with a taxed liver quick to becoming irritable and inflammatory. This is important to examine as all acne is related to the Pitta dosha.

Because Pitta also governs the blood, in Ayurveda acne vulgaris is a rakta disorder (the cellular matter in the blood). Cleansing the blood system is key to clarifying the skin.

Hormones

Hormones are a common cause of breakouts. Many women get them around their menstruation period, as it is a high candida time. Others experience this coming off the birth-control pill when their bodies are trying to rebalance. Any hormonal changes or imbalances may result in pimples and cause excessive heat. That being said, it is important not to feel that hormonal-related blemishes are inevitable. Many assume that they cannot change their hormonal patterns, but with the help of a knowledgeable alternative health practitioner or physician, we can rebalance our bodies and hormones.

When we think of the link between hormones and blemishes, we often think of puberty and its influence on teenaged acne. But it may not simply be hormonal fluctuations which are causing this condition. During puberty, the changing body is under considerable stress. It uses a lot of pantothenic acid at this time, as well as during pregnancy and breast-feeding.

Holistic dermatologist, Dr. Lit-Hung Leung, caused controversy when he stated that, without ample pantothenic acid (Vitamin B5) coenzyme A, fatty acids do not get metabolized and become oil in the skin instead. Therefore Dr. Leung recommends high doses of pantothenic acid as a natural way to treat acne.

It was a client who educated me about Dr. Leung as she found his methods effective in treating her severe acne problem.

Stress

Stress taxes the whole body, lowering its immune system, causing it to dehydrate, leaving it defenseless to bacteria and infection, and decreasing its ability to regenerate. As previously discussed, stress imbalances hormones causing acne.

Constipation

One client, with whom I'd been working for three years, had such congested skin that she would not go anywhere without makeup. When I did extractions, it seemed almost as if every pore was clogged. For most facials, I allot fifteen minutes or so for extractions, but hers were taking me well over an hour. When she returned for follow-up treatments, every pore would again be full of dried sebum. We tried many different approaches, but her skin would clear up for only a few weeks before yet another severe breakout. We could never stabilize her, and I simply could not understand it. She was a holistic nutrition student, with an excellent diet; she drank three liters of water per day, and exercised regularly. We tried to track her stress levels, and did frequent facials with only minimal results. Finally, I asked her how many times per day she eliminated, stating that twice was ideal.

"Really? I'm lucky if I have a bowel movement every two or three days!" she exclaimed.

With such a back up of toxicity in her body, no wonder she was eliminating through her skin. I had assumed she had regular bowel movements because she was so educated about food and the body, and I was shocked to hear how constipated her bowels were.

I recommended she take a tincture of milk thistle for her liver, and to drink a half-cup of aloe vera juice with water twice per day. This cools Pitta and is a mild laxative. I also prescribed a fiber-based laxative.

Amazingly, after about a month, her skin looked smooth and clear. I was sure she must have resorted to taking severe antibiotics or the birth-control pill, but she announced with a smile, "I've done only what you told me to do, and I'm not even wearing makeup. You changed my life!"

An obvious sign of constipation is an abundance of blackheads on the jaw line and lower cheeks – just remember, if you do not release toxins through the bowels, they will come out through your skin.

What Your Blemishes are Telling You

The affected areas of the face and the type of acne, will indicate what is happening inside the body. This can be an early-warning sign of illness and organ dysfunction. Often this is a blessing in disguise, though we rarely see acne that way. (Refer to the face-mapping section).

Types of Acne

Comedones

Comedones are whiteheads and blackheads, also called "non-inflammatory acne."

Whiteheads occur when sebum and bacteria are trapped below the skin's surface. They may be virtually invisible or appear as white bumps. Blackheads occur when the trapped sebum and bacteria are partially open to the skin's surface. Because of oxidization of the skin's melanin, they become black in color.

These are Vata blemishes which usually accumulate from dehydration and often cluster in areas with thinner skin. Treating this type of acne is usually simply done by applying a richer moisturizer and eating moist foods to soften stools. Since these blemishes may be from toxins within the colon, also related to Vata, constipation should always be considered.

Papules

Papules and pustules are more severe on the continuum. These Pitta-type blemishes are categorized as inflammatory acne. They are red and agitated bumps on the skin. They do not come to a head and are usually smaller than pustules. Since all inflammation and infection is related to heat, balancing Pitta is important. Cooling and calming is commonly done with sandalwood, amalaki and coconut oil.

Since this acne is stress-related, cooling the diet and angry emotions is also important for treating holistically. Breathing exercises can be particularly beneficial. Through yoga, Ayurveda offers an umbrella of exercises for healing. Pranayama (controlled breath) and meditation are fantastic for stress-related blemishes.

Pustules

These are red, inflamed pimples with a white, puss-filled head. They need an anti-bacterial treatment for prevention. Extracting them, when they are ready, is the fastest way to heal them. If it is not possible to see a professional, try a drying clay or mud spot treatment. This helps dry and draw out the blemish so we do not need to extract it. While the presence of pus indicates a bacterial infection related to Pitta, an abundance of fluid is associated with Kapha.

Cystic Acne (also known as Blind Pimples)

These large, often tender pimples have no white head. They are deep, long-lasting blemishes which lie beneath the skin and are sometimes not visible. They can be removed by pricking them with a needle and extracting its fluid. This should only be done by a professional because cystic acne scars very easily.

Applying arnica helps to drain the fluid because arnica promotes circulation. Unlike most acne, cystic acne is governed primarily by Kapha (water-accumulation and retention). It is usually found on the chin or jaw line and most often is related to hormonal imbalance.

Balancing Kapha is important, as is topical antibacterial action. Cystic acne is the only type of acne that requires oil-reduction on the skin's surface, along with bacteria-killing, heating herbs. Decreasing oily foods, along with a routine of vigorous exercise to move the lymphatic fluid, are good for preventing cysts.

Because cystic acne occurs after infection has attacked the dermis layer of the skin, treatments which work on that layer are needed. Some say severe cases require antibiotics. I always advocate the avoidance of internal medication, but each of us must use the treatment which aligns with our own personal needs, values and expectations.

Parts of the Face and What They Mean

If acne is product-related, it will generally be dispersed all over the face. When isolated to specific areas, it indicates an internal problem.

If you refer back to the face map, you will see the correspondence between facial areas and internal organs. In Ayurveda, Vata governs the top of the face, Pitta the middle (eyes to upper lip) and Kapha, the lower part. This means that where there is acne, one must balance that dosha.

Allergic breakouts on the upper cheeks relate to the lungs – those who quit smoking may also break out here, as toxins are being purged after being suppressed. The chin is hormonal – those stopping the birth-control pill may experience breakouts here. The forehead is related to the colon, the lymphatic system and an overactive mind. The jaw line indicates sluggishness, constipation and hormonal imbalance.

Conventional Solutions and Why They Do Not Work

Many panicked teenagers seek the advice of dermatologists at the first sight of blemishes. The popular solution is to dry the skin with salicylic acid and benzoyl peroxide, or peel it with harsh retinol creams. This only worsens the problem by unbalancing and depleting the skin, causing more blemishes. Stripping also leaves the skin more susceptible to infection and, therefore, acne. The next step is usually a more powerful one: antibiotics, birth-control pills and retinoid Accutane.

I, myself, took antibiotics for teenage acne. While my skin cleared up, it was blotchy, dry, flaky and very sensitive. I also felt nauseous. But when I stopped taking this medication, my face was the worst it had ever been. Many of my acne clients have had the same experience. They come to me in terrible condition after stopping the birth-control pill, since such drugs and chemicals are a short-term solution, producing worse aftereffects.

Antibiotics

Antibiotics also dehydrate the internal organs and cause photosensitivity. This is what happened to me, and is now taking years to repair. Since adult acne is usually liver-related, when these sufferers take medications they run the risk of further damaging their already dysfunctional livers for temporary solutions.

Birth-control pills

Birth-control pills are a drastic acne solution, since artificially altering hormone levels is harmful to both the skin and our overall health. Also, results are only sustained if we keep taking them, once we stop our acne will return.

Accutane

Currently, the most popular, aggressive, internal medication is Accutane. Side-effects include dry skin, constipation, vaginal dryness, inflammation of the liver, gene damage and dehydration of the internal organs. This treatment is especially popular among males, possibly because their acne becomes severe so quickly due to testosterone and lack of education about skincare.

Accutane has also been linked with more than 1,300 psychiatric side-effects, including severe depression, and has been cited as the cause of more than 66 suicides. While very results-oriented, it is holistically unhealthy, and the damage can be long-lasting.

More Natural Solutions

Acne: Not a War

Most people view acne as an enemy. Seeing a pimple on their face makes them want to eliminate it, extract it, and dry it out. This reflects the attitude that acne is a topical and external problem, not an internal imbalance expressing itself.

After years of thinking and behaving this way, I realized that I needed to be kinder to my skin. I started making it healthier as opposed to damaging or depleting it. Only then was my skin able to heal itself and repair my complexion.

Simple Rules for Banishing Blemishes

1. **Use natural skincare products.** Do not clog pores with petroleum-based products that sit on the skin's surface. Most of us acne-sufferers do not need harsh, drying cleansers and creams. The best routine includes chemical-free makeup, gentle cleansers and healing moisturizers.
2. **Do not be afraid of oil.** The absence of oil on the surface of the skin promotes the body to produce oil to compensate. Our bodies are always trying to balance themselves, and not using a moisturizer in a cold, dry environment can create an even bigger oil problem.
3. **Do not get too stressed about your blemishes.** Some say stress causes break outs as it uses up Vitamin B5. Some say it dehydrates the skin, and that dehydration causes acne. Others say stress lowers the immune system, making the body more vulnerable to acne. Whatever your school of thought, stress contributes to blemish-prone skin.
4. **Good skin is based on wellness.** An acne solution should not be negative for the body as a whole. If skin looks unattractive, there are often underlying health issues to address. Often a weak liver causes acne by preventing toxins from being filtered out so that the body must find another avenue to eliminate waste. Detoxify the liver and avoid Accutane.
5. **Take care of your lifestyle and diet.** Eat lots of fresh vegetables and drink two liters of water per day. This cleanses our system and hydrates our cells. As I became more hydrated, not only did my skin clear up, but it became moister, less sensitive and less irritated.

Rosacea, Eczema, Sensitive and Allergic Skin

Sensitive Skin: Seeing Red!

Sensitive skin types react to internal or external stimulation with redness, blemishes and dermatitis. Whether it is simple flushing or an allergic rash, the root cause is stimulation of the vascular system.

Causes of Sensitivity

Genetics

Dermatologists commonly blame genetics for sensitivity and rosacea. I dislike simply faulting genetic factors because it positions us to believe that our sensitivity is unavoidable. While we may have a genetic predisposition to a more stimulated cardiovascular system and rosacea-prone skin color, we can control inflammation by correcting its cause and balancing our bodies.

Cardiovascular System

Those of us who have inherited a more stimulated cardiovascular system (a tendency toward high blood pressure, high Pitta, poor digestion and allergies) tend to have a more surging blood flow and capillary dilation, causing breakage and redness. This is the reason for blushing, which may be constant or acute, depending on the stimulation of the cardiovascular system. This is another reason why skin hydration is important – to keep the capillaries flexible and prevent their damage.

Skin Colour

Our genetic makeup dictates the melanin in our skin, and melanin can make sensitivity more or less visible. Though fair complexions appear to have a greater tendency to redness, this has more to do with dehydration, or skin thinness than colour. Lighter skin actually has less melanin and therefore a lessened immune response to stimulus. While melanin provides darker skin with more protection from the sun, it is actually more reactive because of the heightened immune response. This causes hyper-pigmentation and inflammation even though irritation is less noticeable in these pigmented skin types.

The Environment

Sensitivity is accentuated by heat and trauma. The following are environmental (external) factors which contribute to rosacea, eczema, allergic and sensitive skin.

Overexposure to Sun

Heating or burning of the skin causes inflammation and damages cells. This also causes long-term dehydration. Remember, we previously discussed how sun exposure relates to acne-prone skin. Because acne is a form of inflammation, the same reasons that sun causes blemishes apply to sensitivity.

Diet

Alcohol, tobacco, caffeine, spicy foods, fried foods, over-cooked and barbequed foods cause dehydration and capillary dilation which will worsen sensitivity. Pitta-increasing diets will aggravate sensitivity while a Pitta-pacifying diet will soothe and calm redness. Refer to an Ayurvedic food chart for more details.

Lifestyle

A high-stress life overburdens the circulatory system causing chronic high blood pressure and vessel dilation.

The Elements

Any trauma will contribute to sensitivity. Wind and pollution exposure deplete and damage the skin on a cellular level.

Extreme temperatures and fluctuations can damage and break capillaries leading to chronic redness. Following the advice in the "Protect Yourself "section is essential.

Dehydration

Dehydration is always present when dealing with sensitivity as it weakens the skin's barrier function. Think of the skin as a brick wall: The cells, like bricks, create a dense barrier, along with the intracellular lipids which function like mortar. When skin cells dehydrate, they shrink, causing tiny spaces or cracks in the wall. These create weakness, making it easier for bacteria, infection and other environmental pollutants to infiltrate, and for moisture to escape from the deeper cells.

Hydration levels also genetically determine sensitivity. Asian skin has a tendency to experience more transepidermal water-loss making it more sensitive. Hyper-pigmentation occurs when dehydration allows skin to be constantly irritated.

Moisture always calms the skin, and hydrated skin has the capacity to regenerate and heal itself.

Pitta Imbalance/ Emotional Stress

Those with rosacea and sensitive skin are often individuals who put a lot of pressure on themselves, who have repressed anger and frustration, and who are militant perfectionists. These characteristics heighten the heart rate and produce internal heat.

According to Ayurveda, Pitta's tendency to compete, organize and become agitated also cause the stress that stimulates the cardiovascular system. All inflammation is governed by Pitta (fire).

Calming the mind, channeling energies, eating lighter foods such as salads and avoiding spicy foods are recommended. So are using cooling essential oils, such as jojoba, coconut and sandalwood.

Couperose

Couperose refers to dilated blood vessels. The term refers to poor elasticity of the capillary wall.

All rosacea, sensitivity and broken capillaries include couperose.

Skincare for those who are Sensitive

Some sensitivity is self-induced. When I had acne, I inflicted harm on my skin through the use of glycolic peels and a variety of drying agents which depleted my skin's barrier function and made me photosensitive. Caution is advised when using AHAs, retinols and glycolics. Any skin with visible redness should avoid these types of peels.

Using natural, gentle skincare geared toward calming and soothing is important. However, when using natural ingredients, avoid stimulating herbs and additives such as ginseng, Vitamin C and lemon essential oil.

Cooling and comforting ingredients like sandalwood, chamomile, helichryse, melissa and lavender will lessen redness. Try to use organic products because pesticides and chemical solvents can irritate.

From a more scientific standpoint, collagen and elastin products are fantastic for rebuilding the skin, but finding and using those with a natural base is essential for proper penetration.

Ingredients to Slather On!

- Jojoba oil
- Evening primrose oil
- Coconut oil
- Superoxide dismutase
- Sandalwood
- Chamomile
- Helichryse
- Rose hip
- Melissa
- Vitamin E (tocopheryl acetate)
- Calendula
- Collagen/ elastin

Ingredients to Avoid!

- Benzoyl peroxide
- Salycilic acid
- Ethyl alcohol
- Sodium laurel sulfate
- Petroleum, petrolatum
- Propylene glycol
- High amounts of Ginseng, Vitamin C, Glycolic acid and AHAs, Lemon

Sensitivity and Lymphatic Drainage

When it comes to redness, most of us think primarily about avoiding aggravation to the skin. Some of us will go further by trying to restore its health to prevent inflammation. Only a few of us consider lymphatic congestion and the skin's water-retention to be part of the problem.

Often Kapha people have inflammation on the cheeks. They may also have superficial dehydration due to a lack of circulation. In these cases, blood is not moving freely through the capillaries, and the lymph is not draining. When those with Kapha tendencies or imbalances (prone to congestion and puffiness) swell with lymphatic fluid, pressure is put on the blood vessels, dilating and breaking them. This can be prevalent in the thigh area, creating spider veins, and in other areas where cellulite exists, further cutting off circulation.

Sometimes lymphatic congestion cuts off circulation, causing dehydration and undernourished skin cells.

Lymphatic drainage is a key to soothing sensitive skin. Often I have found pressure-point massage drains off the lymphatic and glandular congestion almost immediately, bringing down redness.

Rosacea

Rosacea is an extreme form of sensitivity. It is a cardiovascular disorder, appearing as reddened skin, possibly with papules and a thickened texture. Rosacea is becoming more common through greater exposure to extreme weather and lifestyle stress.

Rosacea, also known as "acne rosacea," can cause acne-like bumps, which do not come to a head and are full of lymphatic fluid. They can appear chronically, or as flare-ups during times of stress, or in extreme weather.

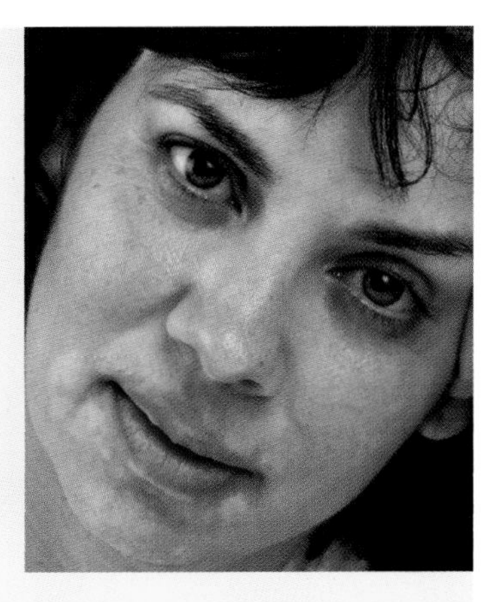

The Four Faces of Rosacea

There are different degrees of severity to rosacea. With care, you can prevent the condition from worsening to its next stage.

Stage 1 – pre-rosacea:
Skin sensitivity with occasional blushing and flushing.
Stage 2 – mild rosacea:
Skin which is highly sensitive and prone to flushing with heated inflammation. Irritation lasts for several hours.
Stage 3 – moderate rosacea:
Permanent redness, easily aggravated into stinging, burning and heated inflammation. Possible papules and the appearance of broken blood vessels.
Stage 4 – severe rosacea:
A minority of rosacea sufferers progress to this stage. Papules, deformation, bulbous nose. Usually occurs in men, often induced by alcoholism.

Causes of Rosacea

Rosacea is always related to the cardiovascular system. This is an extreme Pitta imbalance. Both Eastern and Western medical physicians agree that rosacea sufferers should avoid things which stimulate the heart rate. This includes:

- Spicy food
- Alcohol
- Cigarette smoke
- Cardio exercise
- Stress
- Cardiovascular stimuli
- Emotionally stressful situations
- Extreme heat (dilates capillaries)
- Extreme cold (dilates capillaries)
- Barbecued foods

Other aspects to controlling rosacea is digestion and elimination (Pitta governs digestion). When one of my clients broke out in papulopustular rosacea (rosacea with papules) for the first time, she was so determined to control her skin that she started a series of colon irrigation treatments and eliminated allergens and difficult to digest foods in her diet. The results were impressive. After approximately one year, I could not even tell she had had rosacea. Though it was a struggle, with patience and natural treatments, she attained beautiful, healthy skin without medication.

Treatments for Rosacea: Conventional vs. Holistic

While rosacea varies from client to client in degree of severity, dermatologists tend to treat all cases in the same way. Oral antibiotics, like tetracycline, and topical antibiotics, such as metronidazole (commonly called "Metro Gel"), are popularly prescribed to relieve symptoms. But these solutions are temporary if not counterproductive. While metronidazole can damage skin and even worsen rosacea, antibiotics increase heat. According to Ayurveda, oral antibiotics aggravate Pitta which is also the original cause of rosacea.

Lasers and Intense Pulse Light (IPL) can also be used to eliminate damaged capillaries, but this is purely cosmetic as these treatments do not prevent or treat the root cause of their formation. IPL is best practiced in conjunction with a program of internal healing to produce long-term results.

As with generally sensitive skin, the holistic approach for rosacea must encompass anti-inflammatory lifestyle practices such as stress-management, a soothing skincare regime, a cooling diet (Pitta reducing), and the avoidance of stimulants (ex. tobacco, alcohol and caffeine). Solutions should be specific to the individual. Since rosacea and sensitive skin have multiple causes, a holistic approach appropriately involves the whole body, mind and spirit.

Eczema

Eczema is extremely common, and many people mistaken it for an allergic reaction.

Changes of season can trigger eczema, along with food allergies and skincare products, but these are not the root causes.

Characteristics of Eczema

- Patches of dry, flaky skin.
- Sometimes itchy and hot.
- Sometimes bumps which look like water blisters, indicating infection.
- Often so irritating it awakens you or disturbs sleep during the night.

There are various types of eczema. Understanding them helps to identify and properly aid whichever form is being experienced.

Vata Eczema

Vata eczema is easiest to treat. It is dry, flaky and chapped. The application of a rich cream or pure oil feels wonderful, like a refreshing drink for the skin. It is important to ensure only pure vegetable oils are used as they fully absorb and nourish.

Pitta Eczema

Pitta eczema is inflamed, and this type of eczema often experiences a burning sensation. While it can also be dry and flaky, it is important to avoid straight oils and rich creams because oil will accentuate Pitta's heat. Compare this to frying food – oil makes the pan much hotter. In my personal experience, even cooling oils seem to aggravate Pitta inflammation. Instead, I recommend cooling gels, aloe vera and light lotions. Repeated application may be needed throughout the day to keep the skin moist and support its barrier function. Spraying hydrosols of rose and chamomile can also be very effective.

My own desperation during an eczema outbreak on my face led to the discovery of our bestselling Pitta eczema product. I had been using emollient products which were increasing heat and causing hive-like reactions. Hastily, I applied my Pure + Simple Firming Eye Gel . . . and it was fantastic. Though firming and nourishing to combat aging, it was light in texture for the sensitive eye area with its small pores. Therefore, it provided protection and moisture without heat-inducing oil. After this product was reintroduced as our Skin Softening Moisture Lotion, it became our most popular moisturizer for sensitive skin.

Kapha Eczema

Kapha eczema has a look of wetness, like light perspiration on the skin. This type is at risk of becoming infected by fungus. Often it acquires what looks like water blisters, and it is very itchy. Keep this eczema clean, and use anti-bacterial, anti-fungal herbs on the skin such as tea tree (diluted), peppermint and sage which have purifying properties. Avoid rich, moist products.

What Causes Eczema?

There is no official cause for eczema, but the following are triggers to eczema outbreaks.

Dehydration

Though there is no cited cause, extreme dehydration has been the trigger for every eczema condition I have observed.

Stress

Stress-related breakouts often occur on the insides of elbows and the backs of knees. Post-traumatic stress disorder may also trigger eczema.

Poor Digestion

Those with eczema need a healthy digestive system to absorb hydration. Proper elimination of toxins, candida and parasites is also important.

Parasites

It has been speculated that parasites can cause eczema. When I had my first severe outbreak of eczema a colon therapist who followed the Hulda Clark's electromagnetic method informed me that she thought it was parasite-related.

Imbalance of Internal Elements

Eczema breakouts are most likely to occur during a change of season or of climate when the body is taxed through readjustment. This is often when Kapha blisters appear, usually during transition from a drier to a wetter environment. Vata eczema occurs when going from hotter to colder, drier weather. But climate change is only a trigger, because the external environment brings out our imbalance of internal elements that these symptoms are displayed. Furthermore, the qualities of these symptoms reflect the qualities of the imbalance.

Travel

Constant travel can lead to an eczema condition. I always become inflamed after flying. This is because it causes excess Vata and dehydration. The combination of experiencing a new climate, plus the dry airplane environment and the stress of traveling provide a perfect formula for eczema. Tip: When flying, lubricate your skin, and frequently spray it with a hydrosol to avoid a breakout. Constant flying and traveling ages the skin rapidly.

Conventional vs. Holistic Solutions

The conventional protocol usually prescribes cortisone cream to bring down the appearance of redness. This thins the skin without treating the sources of the imbalance. Treating the appropriate doshas is more effective than any cookie-cutter solution.

Rules to Keep Eczema-Free

1. Avoid alcohol in your skincare as well as in your diet (it is dehydrating).
2. Take omega-3 essential fatty acids. They are fantastic for lubricating the intestines, holding hydration and aiding digestion. Remember, oil is not water-soluble so it will help hold water.
3. Use black mud and dead sea minerals containing sulfur in your skincare. But not all dead sea products are created equal as some use a chemical base which is counterproductive. Martina Gebhardt has a Black Mud Line which is excellent for clearing eczema.
4. Use algae. Algae in our skincare helps us hold moisture without needing to use a heavy emollient.

Hyper-Pigmentation

Taking many forms such as lesions, freckles and uneven skin tone, hyper-pigmentation generally refers to skin discoloration. This is a growing concern in the beauty industry today due to the ever-increasing power of the sun.

The Darkness Explained

Our skin's colour is determined by the amount of melanin it possesses. Melanin (our skin's pigment) is produced by melanocytes, which are found in our skin's epidermis layer. The more active our melanocytes, the darker our skin will be.

Structurally, a melanocyte has been compared to an octopus. Melanocytes contain pod-shaped organelle called melanosomes which hold particles of melanin within them. These pods are created and passed through the octopus-like arms of the melanocytes to the keratinocytes (cells that make up 90 per cent of the epidermis). It is here that they gain colour. When this process becomes over-active, pigmentation is visible. UV rays and other factors cause over/ under-activity of these melanocytes, creating lighter and darker patches.

Keratinocytes have a lifespan of two-to-three weeks. This is interesting when compared to "rogue" melanocytes which can live for multiple years. This demonstrates how long-term a pigmentation issue can persist.

Those of us with sensitive skin are more susceptible to discoloration as redness and inflammation turns brown over time. While UVA and UVB rays promote dysfunction of our melanocytes, the inflammation caused by burning our skin also causes discoloration. Scarring is a classic example of inflammation becoming pigmentation.

Other triggers are trauma, heat, internal problems, diet, medications, topical irritants and improper skincare.

Usually hyper-pigmentation is a gradual process, only becoming visible years after the damage has occurred.

Dehydration and Pigmentation

In my experience, persons with sensitive skin are more prone to pigmentation. Because sensitivity is increased by dehydration, it has also been my observation that pigmented topical moisturization almost instantaneously lessens its darkness. Though the change is not dramatic, this indicates that long-term replenishment can treat hyper-pigmentation.

This has been supported by Dr. Vasant Lad's finding that pigmentation could also be due to a Vata corruption in the rakta dhatu (red blood-cell tissues). While the blood is governed by Pitta, a Vata dysfunction within this Pitta environment can cause the disruption. Calming Vata with the application of rich oils, and cleansing the blood helps treat hyper-pigmentation.

Hormones and Pigmentation

Because melanin production is powered by MSH (Melanocyte Stimulating Hormone), it is no wonder that our hormonal system influences hyper-pigmentation. Adrenal stress, along with estrogen and progesterone, can also contribute. Many pregnant women experience changes in skin color, from pigmentation on their abdomens (stretching and inflammation) to what is known as the "pregnancy mask" on their faces (caused by the hormonal changes of pregnancy).

Pheomelanin and Eumelanin

Western scientists say those with "the redhead gene" are five times more susceptible to freckling and melanoma. This is due to an abundance of pheomelanin (pink skin pigment). Upon UV exposure, pheomelanin produces free radicals. This gene does not necessarily dictate red hair, but just a potential for it in our genetics. Oddly enough, red hair is a Pitta characteristic.

Eumelanin is a black/brown pigment. When we tan, eumelanin absorbs the energy of light without becoming a free radical, thus protecting the skin. Since amino acid, tyrosine, stimulates eumelanin production, many chemical solutions inhibit tyrosine, but once treatments are stopped, the pigmentation returns.

Pigmentation and Skin Colour

Skin colour is often determined by ancestry. Those of us with darker skins come from places where more sun exposure has created a need to protect itself through pigment. This pigment protects the skin from UV rays and is a natural form of SPF. Nevertheless, darker skins easily become discolored after burning because of their active melanocytes, while fairer skins turn red.

Conventional Solutions

Peeling with a retinol or a chemical agent is the most common solution. Naturally-derived lactic acid is one of the best for breaking up pigmentation and for easy penetration, provided it is in a natural base. Lactic acid must be used in conjunction with sun protection, especially when it is in high concentrations.

This does not change the fact that all peels thin and dehydrate the skin while increasing sun-sensitivity. This is obviously counterproductive, since dehydration causes pigmentation, and skin cannot heal when dehydrated. When using a peel, follow with a nourishing, natural moisturizer is essential.

Another conventional solution is bleaching. While effective in inhibiting pigmentation, this can be harsh on sensitive skin and extremely bad for our health. Hydroquinone, a mainstream bleaching agent, has been named as a carcinogen.

Chemical-Free Solutions

Natural solutions are also very beneficial, but expectations must be mitigated. This is true when treating any skin ailment, but especially with pigmentation as it is very difficult to cure completely. Natural solutions will be able to aid the appearance of pigmentation, but not get rid of it completely.

To lighten and prevent darkening, nourishment is essential:

Collagen is fantastic for restoring the skin's moisture levels. It can even fade scars if they are still in their young, red state. The older the pigmentation, the more difficult to diminish.

Oils like borage, rose hip and evening primrose have also been known to help regeneration and to yield excellent results with discoloration. One of my clients told me that the darkness of their pigmented spots have decreased by approximately one third after using rose hip oil daily for three years. While this may not seem dramatic, keep in mind that this form of treatment is without peels or bleaching.

Engaging in a program of gentle repair, while using more technological treatments, is a better option for those with more ambitious expectations.

Intense Pulse Light (IPL)

IPL is extremely effective for diminishing uneven pigmentation (even freckles), but it requires a greater time and financial investment. Light energy stimulates the body to heal itself and increases collagen production. Before treatment, the skin's immunity should be boosted with a calming and cooling regime; afterwards, focus should be placed on adopting a restoring and protective regime.

Light Emitting Diode (LED)

LED therapy is another excellent treatment for pigmentation. This low-intensity light repairs skin and stimulates collagen production. This technology has been used for healing during skin-cancer therapies and provides safe support for your pigmentation program. It is most effective when used after peeling with microdermabrasion or post-IPL therapy.

Internal solutions

Hyper-pigmentation requires us to reduce excess Pitta by cooling the internal body. Remember, all transformation is governed by Pitta. The most effective way is to detoxify Pitta and rebalance the dosha.

Intense Pitta detoxification can be achieved through panchakrama, which means loosening Pitta toxins through oiling the body externally and internally. The process requires oiling and intense sweating for multiple days, followed by purging toxins through laxatives. The oleation ritual brings all excess Pitta toxins to their original site – the small intestine – to be cleared out. Laxatives differ in results, depending on your constitution. Gentle laxatives include castor oil, aloe vera, triphala and prunes. After this, take heating herbs to increase digestive fire to help the skin digest sunlight. This regime is very effective in decreasing pigmentation.

If you do not want to partake in panchakarma, then try eating Pitta-pacifying foods that are sweet, bitter and cooling, while avoiding spicy, sour and oily ones. Detoxifying the liver is also key in clearing away excess Pitta.

Pigmentation Prevention

As always, prevention is the best practice. Year-round sun protection is essential, along with keeping the skin hydrated. Using restorative ingredients, such as collagen, support the skin and boost immunity. As for the rest of our bodies, a strong immune system can prevent disease even when we are in contact with all the causative variables.

Avoid skin trauma. This can be in the form of irritation, burns, allergens and scarring from improper healing.

Though internal prevention is imperative, it is so often overlooked. Avoiding Pitta-aggravating foods and "hot" mindsets are an effective way to maintain beautiful skin.

Restorative Ingredients:

- Collagen
- Elastin
- Manuka Honey
- Borage Oil
- Geranium
- Lavender
- Calendula

Skin tags (benign skin growths) are also a byproduct of excess Pitta (governing transformation, but also involving Kapha accumulation). Often darker in colour, they also disrupt a smooth, even complexion. In these cases, both Pitta and Kapha would need to be decreased in the body.

Skin Aging

We are continuously aging. Many people fear growing older because they do not understand that *aging* is simply *changing.* Stopping this process is a futile goal which is stifling to personal growth.

Aging is just a reminder that our bodies are our vessels, something we cannot fully control. As we move closer to wisdom, we move away from the physical. Our minds expand with life experience, while our bodies degenerate, mirroring a balance which exists in everything. Nevertheless, modern-day demands and expectations also govern us. Our youth-obsessed society motivates us to be proactive, but we must see "anti-aging" as supporting the process of maturation and promoting healthy tissue. For best results, we must not only treat our skin topically, but rejuvenate ourselves inside as well.

The Aging Process

To support or defy anything, we must understand it.

What is Aging?

We generally define aging as a group of symptoms which indicate our bodies have been lived-in. Wrinkles, jowls, loss of tone and age-spots indicate we have stopped developing and are entering the age of experience. It is natural for our tissues to wilt and our systems to become exhausted with activity, but anyone who takes care of body, mind and spirit can evolve gracefully.

With aging, the two facets we must focus on are:

1. Slowed metabolism
2. Inflammation

Slowed Metabolism

As we age our bodies slow down. As mentioned previously, while a 25-year-old's cell turnover occurs approximately every 28 days, a 75-year-old's occurs approximately every 90 days. This is why our skin and body look less youthful and why peeling is the foundation of anti-aging.

It is not only cell turnover which slows, but the healing process. After age 25, there is a drastic drop in our collagen and elastin production, resulting in loss of firmness, tone and hydration.

As we mature, our silhouettes also change and our body fat increases as muscle tone decreases. This is because our metabolism has slowed down, making it more and more apparent that exercise is essential along with a healthy diet. No longer can we ignore those needs as we could in our forgiving and short-sighted youth.

Blockages also accumulate as our whole body's system slows making detoxification and waste removal less rapid. Exercise helps prevent stagnation, which impedes our qi and blood flow. Our skin becomes less nourished, because it is not being fed by blood circulation, and our bodies grow colder, especially our hands and feet.

Acupuncture facials are a recent trend. The results are excellent, based on the dispersing of blockages and the increase in stimulation. General acupuncture is also fantastic as an anti-aging measure.

Inflammation

The other cause of aging is inflammation, an inevitable response to crisis or damage. Through sun-exposure, trauma and stress, we inflame our bodies and tissues, resulting in deterioration in our joints, muscles and skin. As well as creating free radicals, inflammation stretches and breaks the capillaries. It also puts pressure on the skin, producing wrinkles.

A typical diet causes heat and inflammation. Meat is very acidic and hard to digest, inflaming the internal body. Refined sugar has the same effect, leading many experts to conclude it causes wrinkles. Age-spots are another result of too much sugar as the body tries to expel simple carbohydrates. Because of this overload, fat blocks melanin, dispersing pigment in an uneven pattern.

Many women experience a lot of inflammation because of hormonal changes, creating an imbalance. This is especially true during perimenopause.

Menopause

Menopause causes drastic changes in women's bodies as we pass from our child-bearing stage into more reflective years.

Many women see this change as depressing. It becomes increasingly difficult to maintain youthful-looking skin as estrogen levels drop, decreasing tone and suppleness. This absence of estrogen also lets the testosterone hormone flourish, causing excess hair growth on the upper lip and chin. I suggest that, instead of experiencing change as a diminishing of beauty, we celebrate it as a transition.

According to Ayurveda, this is Vata time (a joint in time, a change). This means women may experience Vata-dysfunction characteristics: scattered mental patterns, forgetfulness, oversensitivity to our surroundings and insomnia. Vata physicality increases: roughness and thinning of the skin and hair, frailness, dullness and dryness as well as brittleness of the bones.

It is also during this transition that other dosha imbalances become more obvious.

Those with high Pitta will experience hot flashes, breakouts and mood fluctuations while those with Kapha accumulation will experience water-retention and lethargy.

With the dramatic decrease in estrogen, osteoporosis becomes a concern, as estrogen facilitates the bone's absorption of calcium from the blood and inhibits its loss. According to Ayurveda, this is caused by high Vata.

Asthi agni (governing the bone tissue) increases as the body tries to compensate for estrogen decrease. Shatavari is an excellent herb to take for natural estrogen. Synthetic hormone-replacement therapy can increase Pitta. During menopause, we should calm our Vata and support this beautiful time of transformation.

Tips for an Effortless Transition:

1. **Oil your body every day.** Sesame oil is best for pacifying Vata. Pay special attention to the scalp as this will treat the nervous system.

2. **Relax in a steam room or wet sauna.** This will help moisten Vata, lubricate your body and calm your mind.

3. **Indulge in a monthly facial.** Add a Sea-salt Microdermabrasion treatment. The abrasion will force new skin to the surface, preparing it for deep absorption of a rich moisturizer or nurturing oil.

4. **Use an oil-rich moisturizer** to protect and compensate for lower sebum production. Consider a pure face-oil. Evening primrose is especially good for menopause.

5. **Use a moisturizer or serum** containing hyaluronic acid to compensate for its decrease caused by loss of estrogen.

6. **Go to bed early.** Rest supports any transition. Be careful not to oversleep or to sleep during the day.

7. **Eat moist, grounding foods.** Watery stews and hearty vegetables will help keep the GI tract moist.

8. **Eat foods with estrogenic properties.** This includes spices like turmeric, oregano and thyme, whole-grain cereals, soy and flaxseed.

9. **Protect the kidneys.** In TCM, they influence growth, development and reproduction, making them very important during puberty and menopause (when kidney qi is exhausted). Kidneys are governed by Vata, so they are vulnerable during this time. Monitor your water intake, keep the lower and middle back warm, and avoid excess salt.

10. **Meditate and welcome the change.**

Youth and Aging: the Players

Now that we have outlined causes for signs of aging, we should also discuss how tissues and skin cells are affected.

Collagen

When the subject of anti-aging is discussed, collagen will always be mentioned. Collagen is a protein which makes up most of the cutaneous layer of the skin and the fibres of other connective tissues. It is composed of three chain-links of twisted polypeptides, each of which contains approximately one hundred amino acid units, arranged in a defined sequence.

The skin is composed of five per cent elastin and seventy per cent collagen, making it an ingredient that we cannot overlook. The drastic drop in collagen production in our mid-twenties is just another indication of the slowing of the metabolism.

With aging, collagen also loses its suppleness and its cross-links with other collagen strands, becoming rigid as the structures harden. With this rigidity, the skin also loses its pliability.

Maturation is not the only factor which breaks down collagen. Estrogen does as well, making cells more vulnerable to inflammation. This means birth-control pills and other hormonal medications play a role in collagen's condition.

Excess estrogen can result in the thinning of the skin and contribute to water-retention. It also affects cellulite. Conversely, estrogen improves the skin's texture, making it smoother, moister and firmer due to an increase of hyaluronic acid. It is hyaluronic acid which strengthens the skin's resistance to stretching, increasing its softness and resilience. The use of estrogen in anti-aging skincare, post-menopause, is still being explored.

Elastin

Elastin, making up five per cent of the skin, is the protein responsible for its elasticity. A lack of elastin causes loss of tone and promotes stretch marks.

Elastin is a lighter molecule than collagen, which it supports, and has a web-like structure which weaves in and out, binding collagen's strands. This determines firmness through its tightness or laxness.

As we mature, elastin calcifies and loses its flexibility. Sagging or loose skin is caused by elastase (an agent which breaks it down). Inflammation stimulates elastase production. Beans and soy are elastase inhibitors making them excellent anti-aging foods. Soy oil is an especially beneficial skincare additive.

Stretch Marks are also linked to high blood sugar (remember, sugars cause inflammation).

Free Radicals and Skin Damage

Free radicals are a major factor in aging. They damage cell membranes, phospholipids, proteins and DNA, and cause pigmented lesions. They are produced by pollution, smoking, stress, adrenal breakdown, UV exposure and irritation. Free radicals are essentially a product of inflammation.

They also cause what is referred to as "smoker's skin" by breaking down fatty acids, forming lipofuscin. Lipofuscin gives the skin a yellow hue.

Antioxidants: Free Radical Fighters

- Vitamin E quenches hydroxyl.
- Beta carotene (pre Vitamin A) quenches singlet oxygen.
- Vitamin C regenerates Vitamin E and reacts directly with other ROS.
- Superoxide dimustase
- Catalase
- Green Tea

What are Free Radicals?

Free radicals are atoms or molecules with one or more unpaired electron. Because oxygen (O_2) has two unpaired electrons, it is very reactive with free radicals. While most oxygen in the body is broken down and used to produce energy, the little which is leftover causes chaos in the body.

Superoxide

Superoxide is a free radical formed by UV radiation and some enzyme reactions. Inflammation and sunburn produce it.

Superoxide is known to attack enzymes and cell membranes, causing them to break down. Since a cell's membrane governs what passes in and out, superoxide alters this function. Superoxide is also part of the creation of other free radicals, and when it reacts with itself it creates hydrogen peroxide. While hydrogen peroxide is not a free radical or dangerous on its own, it easily penetrates cell and nuclear membranes and converts to hydroxyl radicals in the presence of iron. Hydroxyl radicals react with DNA, causing serious damage. The DNA becomes abnormal and denatured and cannot function.

Hydroxyl Radicals

These free radicals are very reactive with lipids, enzymes, carbohydrates and proteins, once again causing serious damage and making them one of the biggest players in aging. With free radicals like hydroxyl radical in our bodies, the role of antioxidants is so important.

Vitamin E is an antioxidant which quenches and neutralizes hydroxyl radicals; Vitamin C regenerates Vitamin E. The antioxidant superoxide dismutase also checks them by converting superoxides to peroxide and oxygen. The enzyme catalase then converts the hydrogen peroxide to water and oxygen, preventing production of hydroxyl radicals.

Singlet Oxygen

Singlet oxygen is another common free radical. Singlet oxygen is produced when O_2 has elevated energy. If energy from UV or even fluorescent light is absorbed by O_2, singlet oxygen is created.

When exposed to UV rays, our skin must deal with singlet oxygen. While our body usually overcomes this attack, when its antioxidant defense is overwhelmed, tissue damage results.

Vitamin E, uric acid, beta carotene and biquinone fight singlet oxygen.

Skin through the Ages

Often clients ask me how their skin looks for their age. This is a very difficult question to answer as there is no official way our skin should look at each age, but the following attempts to outline which signs of aging start to become visible at which age.

Skin at age 20

Optimum era for the skin! Now is the time to take care for the future.

Skin at age 30

Due to the drop in collagen production at age 25, first signs of aging start in the 30s: Bone structure defines and frown lines become apparent. Stress in our 30s can cause adult acne. Metabolism slows. Collagen and elastin weakens.

Skin at age 40

Genetic factors kick in. Sun damage done in earlier years finally emerges causing uneven texture and pigmentation. Eye bags, loss of tone and wrinkle rings appear around the neck.

Skin at age 50

Liver/ age-spots form on the skin. The skin looks thinned and firmness is dramatically depleted. Menopause causes hormonal fluctuations. While it can result in breakouts and heat fluctuations, it also produces hyaluronic acid which helps the skin hold hydration. Skin is often dehydrated in this age bracket.

A Summary: Characteristics as the Skin Ages

- Skin susceptible to broken capillaries.
- Sense of touch is dulled.
- Complexion is paler due to poor circulation.
- Less oil/ sebum is produced; therefore, a loss of moisture and less protection.
- Skin is drier and, therefore, more sensitive.
- Collagen and elastin are weakened and production diminishes.
- Sun damage and pigmentation appears.

Conscious beauty

I personally feel that any anti-aging solution must include goals. Goals provide expectations as well as limitations and boundaries. While a plan can be as simple as home-care tailored to the individual, some may desire the results of more extreme treatments. Each plan-of-action must outline how much energy, effort and money is to be invested. Naturally, better results often require a greater investment. Extreme treatments may also be more painful, requiring proper pre- and post-therapy.

Remember that skincare should be practiced with a view to the overall health of the body and mind. Because health is beauty, nurturing one's self is an anti-aging procedure. The choice between an intense treatment protocol or a simple regime depends on personal values and goals.

Treatment Solutions

Because of our society's demand, anti-aging technology is advancing so rapidly that we industry professionals can hardly keep up. Some technology has been derived from the military's research and development: combating the clock in the most literal sense of the term.

Most Popular Treatments Available

Botulinum Toxin/ Botox

Botox has made a splash in the last five years due to its fantastic results. But while it increases in popularity, remember that it is derived from botulinum toxin A, a poisonous bacterium that can cause death in large doses. In fact, botulinum toxin A is arguably one of the most toxic substances in existence. Since the point between our brows are related to the liver according to TCM, Botox injections here can compromise our internal health. Botox is a superficial cover-up to an underlying problem. It is also abnormal for us to think that paralyzing our facial muscles to temporarily stop producing wrinkles is a good solution. Some women in their twenties and thirties are even getting preventative botox. Not only is this bad for our health, but it reflects how vanity has taken priority over the value of our own wellbeing.

Fillers

Injected fillers are another way to treat wrinkles. Since the injectable sector of the beauty industry is always being updated, we must do a lot of research before choosing this option. And while some injections come from human tissue, other fillers which claim to be natural come from cows (bovine collagen) and birds (avian). We must assess these ingredients before permitting their injection into our faces and bodies. Side-effects can include an allergic reaction, the appearance of lumpiness and clumpiness, infection, and our bodies' rejection of the injectable. Some of my clients have had Restylene injections in their lips which resulted in uneven lumps. Fillers are temporary and, like botox, must be done habitually to maintain results. TCM believes that deep peels affect our overall immune systems, and while the cosmetic market regards injections as safe, they are far more invasive than peels.

Surgery

Facelifts and other cosmetic enhancements are a more extreme option, but not one I overlook. While these traumatize the skin, the decision comes back to each individual's expectations and goals. Even some of our more natural-focused clients at Pure + Simple have chosen to undertake them for their own personal reasons. When they do, I stress a pre- and post-procedure program. Keep in mind that incisions to the capillaries and nerve endings, involved in facelifting, impede circulation. After the capillary network has been cut, full restoration is no longer perfectly attainable, often leaving the skin dull and sallow.

Peels

Peels are an excellent way to combat fine lines and dull skin. As already mentioned, I consider peels as successful tactics for keeping skin bright and youthful. However, intense, very deep peels can have a negative affect on our overall health, and may require lengthy recovery time. Because TCM teaches that simple tuina (massage) on the face affects the internal organs as indicated by face-mapping, it is not surprising that TCM also believes that deep peels compromise our immune systems. I am referring to intensive peels which must be done by a professional, and which can take up to five days or more to repair. Opting for deep peels or for gentler, daily peeling treatments, depends on skin types and the results expected. Sea-salt Microdermabrasion is a controlled peeling which can go deeper on problem areas while performing a gentler abrasion on sensitive areas. It also promotes collagen and elastin production. Whatever the choice of peel, it is imperative that each be followed with rich, moisturizing protection. Without this, the newly peeled skin will dehydrate when exposed to the elements.

Lasers

Lasers are a very powerful therapy using light to penetrate 2940nm (nanometers) or more into the skin. This is deep in comparison to other light treatments on the market. They are very effective in rejuvenating, resurfacing and correcting skin imperfections. These aggressive treatments work on and below the skin to modify its architecture, healing sun-damage and increasing collagen content. Plasma lasers are quite intense and painful – a 20-minute treatment requires several days to recover. Pixilated or fractionated lasers are less intense, but do not have the same dramatic lifting. As mentioned before, this market sector is advancing so rapidly that it is important to research the latest options when considering this route.

Photofacials (IPL)

IPL Photofacials use Intense Pulsed Light (with a penetration of 560nm to 1064nm) to promote collagen and elastin production. Treatments may be uncomfortable, but not unbearable, and results can be impressive. Because IPL offers variation in spot-size, beams, time between pulses, etc., this treatment offers much versatility. Photofacials are good for fine lines and toning, but not as effective for very deep lines. I remember going to a seminar on light therapy and medical esthetics in which the speaker advocated deep lines be treated with Botox paired with a filler, while the rest of the skin be rejuvenated with IPL. Though this may be effective, it is a grocery cart of procedures being done to our precious faces. I have found that IPL alone can clear pigmented lesions and broken capillaries to provide a glowing complexion, and I have not yet seen any unhealthy effects. You must protect the skin from the sun before and after IPL treatments, and a series is also necessary for desired results. The number of treatments would depend on the advancement of the problem being treated, the nature of our skin and how proactive we want to be in attaining our goals. While IPL may require more treatments than laser, and at a lesser intensity, I always advocate a more cautious, gradual approach.

Light Emitting Diode (LED)

LED is less intense than IPL and is excellent for wound-healing. Many machines emphasize different lights for different functions (i.e. to kill bacteria, increase collagen production) and a tailored program is required. LED panels are more effective than hand-held devices as they provide more energy.

Endermologie

Endermologie is a face treatment involving manual stimulation to regenerate collagen, elastin and connective tissue. The first step is lymphatic drainage, which is excellent for taking down inflammation, thus lessening puffiness and edema (water-retention); however, results are subtle and will not fulfill the expectations of a facelift.

Cosmetic Acupuncture

Acupuncture is wonderful as a cosmetic treatment because it is results-oriented and holistic. Using the meridians and points of the body to stimulate energy flow is a great way to aid total body health as well as to promote a more youthful complexion. Cosmetic acupuncture stimulates collagen and elastin, removes blockages and treats the internal organs.

Non-Surgical Facelifts

The non-surgical facelift uses electrodes/electronic currents to stimulate and tone our facial muscles. This treatment, which has received much exposure due to celebrity testimonials, is a great, non-invasive way to treat sagging skin and jowls; however, these treatments are only effective in a series and can only aid primitive signs of aging.

Anti-Aging and the Three Principles

The Holistic Approach

To enjoy the natural process of maturation, we must preserve healthy minds and bodies, including glowing skin, by following the three fundamentals I have touched upon throughout this book – moving, purging and nourishing.

1. Moving

Moving: exercise, circulation, metabolism, digestion (physical and emotional), energy flow, transformation.

Since we are composed of energy, movement inside and out is a vital part of our lives. When we do not move, our bodies become deadened, stiff and devitalized. Movement keeps us young.

Energy flow is a fundamental principle of Eastern medicine. TCM uses acupuncture to remove blockages in order to promote the flow of the invisible energy known as qi. Similarly, Reiki, developed in Japan, uses touch to circulate energy. According to Ayurveda, stagnation in the flow of qi is the root of disease. Stagnant physical systems, stagnant thoughts and stagnant emotions cause toxic buildup in our tissues. Instead of flexibility, there is physical rigidity. We also refer to obstacles in our lives as mental blocks. This concept of blockage – an inability to move through or beyond a problem – is so common that we often accept it as normal.

A lack of blood flow in the skin causes dehydration and dullness as our blood transports waste, oxygen and nutrients. This factor is very important, and circulation also determines body heat. Cold or dryness in our hands, feet and face is usually a result of poor circulation even when the core of the body does not seem as affected. Cellulite also results from poor circulation that allows for an accumulation of toxins and water in our fat cells. These bloated cells, which cause dimpling, are not only unsightly to most people, but they also further slow circulation.

Physical exercise not only maintains muscles and keeps the body supple, but it also reduces fatty deposits and activates the bowels, detoxifying the whole system. Movement improves the tone and quality of our muscle tissue. Exercising also causes us to intake more oxygen, which is very cleansing and nourishing and aids in draining the lymph.

Massage is excellent for moving toxins, breaking down blockages and promoting energy flow. Facial exercises firm the muscles that support the skin. Upward massage movements lift the complexion and tones facial muscles, as well as promotes collagen and elastin production. If you use a vegetable-based oil, massage will help it absorb deeply and more quickly.

Facial acupuncture and non-surgical facelifts are effective anti-aging methods because they involve movement. Even light-based therapies (IPL and laser) use energy for stimulation. Encouraging movement in all aspects of our lives can be challenging. It is so easy to fall into habits that overlook the importance of change leading to transformation, but movement is energy, and energy is life force.

2. Purging

Purging: detoxifying, cleansing, shedding, decongesting, exfoliating, eliminating, clearing heat.

Purging is a natural part of life. Our bodies are constantly ridding themselves of toxins and wastes to make way for rebuilding and regrowth. Without this cycle of renewal we cannot survive.

North America has recently become obsessed with detoxification. Fasting, flushing and colon therapy are now so mainstream that they are almost glamorous. But we must maintain balance. While many think of purging in terms of excessive use of laxatives or vomiting, the Pure + Simple concept is simply defined as *eliminating*. Our philosophy is also only to do so gently. We recognize that over-washing and over-exfoliating can be counterproductive and that it is essential not to get too preoccupied or obsessive about cleansing programs.

This detoxification and elimination of waste is also mental and emotional. Purging negative feelings and past experiences, along with too much ego, is important to health. Often people think of their thoughts as separate from their bodies, but blockages in our mental selves manifest in our physical selves. When stress causes hair loss, or embarrassment causes blushing, we see directly how our mental state influences how we look. Therefore, detoxifying the mind can help keep us healthy and astute. Even the act of throwing away possessions and clearing out closet-clutter is therapeutic.

Purging in anti-aging is most commonly through face-peeling. While it can give fantastic results, I personally have always questioned the more aggressive forms. If inflammation causes signs of aging, how can something which wounds the skin be good? And peeling also makes us more vulnerable to UV exposure, contributing to the production of free radicals. This is why I always insist on nourishing, hydrating and soothing the skin when peeling is undertaken. The skin cannot heal without support to compensate for the inflammation caused by the peel. Lymph drainage is another anti-aging practice. Draining the lymph alleviates inflammation and releases cellular toxins by decreasing pressure on the capillaries and inflammation on the skin's surface. It is also excellent in assisting weight loss, along with purging actions of sweating and bowel elimination.

3. Nourishing

Nourishing: feeding, protecting, healing, regenerating, rebuilding, nurturing, replenishing.

That we need to nourish ourselves to stay youthful and vibrant is obvious. With the vitamin and supplement industry booming, we are constantly reminded by the media, as well as our own bodies, what we should replenish to keep healthy. Food, whether for our bodies, our minds or our souls, is the fuel we need to function.

Hydration and moisturizing is how the cosmetic industry promotes nourishing the skin. Water content of the stratum corneum (top layer of the epidermis) is what dictates a youthful appearance. Because the environment is less humid than our bodies, the laws of balancing hypertonic and hypotonic solutions dictate that water will constantly travel from the deeper layers of the epidermis to its outer layers where it will evaporate as perspiration. The water content of the stratum corneum depends on the amount that is being transferred. This is why it is so important to nourish. We can put water inside the skin by hydrating our bodies internally, but supporting the skin externally with proper care is also essential.

Protecting and shielding is another way we nurture ourselves. We cannot heal without a safe environment and if our skin is constantly under siege. In this state of vulnerability, we are unable to regenerate.

Nourishing is not just about consuming or applying the right nutrients. It is also about nurturing ourselves. I firmly believe this should include treatments that pamper us emotionally as well as physically. Because we are tactile beings, it is so beautiful to use touch to connect, center and treat one another. Even the act of choosing to receive a therapy indicates a desire to love the self.

To truly be nourished, we must use products with natural ingredients. Because of the powerful presence of free radicals in our stressful, polluted, ozone-depleted age, antioxidants are a vital new discovery, not merely a cosmetic fad.

It is also important for us to eat foods uncontaminated with synthetic preservatives or toxic pesticides. Food is not simply for sustenance but also for growth. Healthy bodies will actually reject artificial ingredients because they are natural barometers of how we should nourish ourselves. This is equally true of our skin. Because pure, natural products do not contain toxic, clogging ingredients, they can penetrate more deeply and therefore truly revitalize.

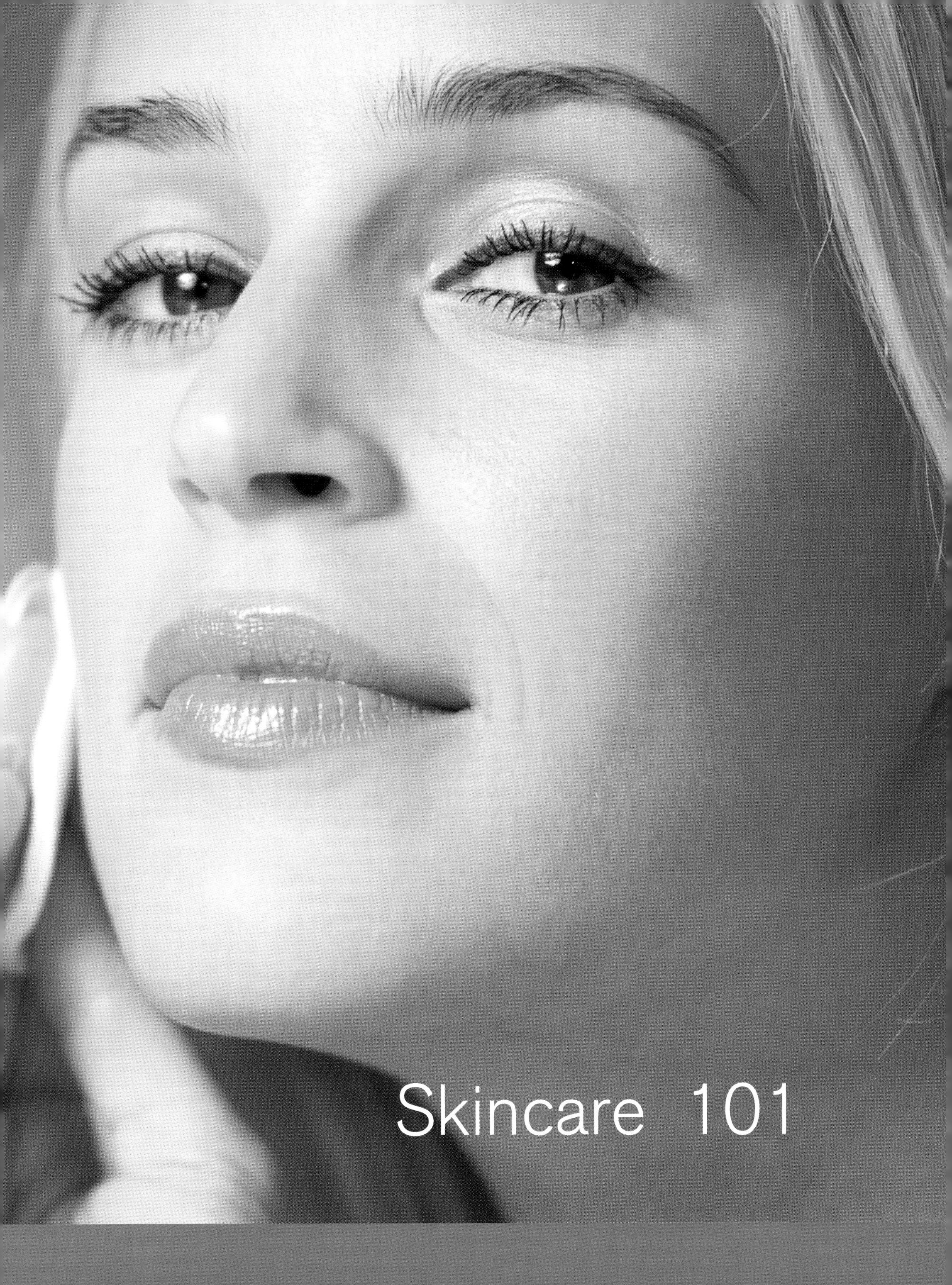

Skincare 101

CHAPTER 12

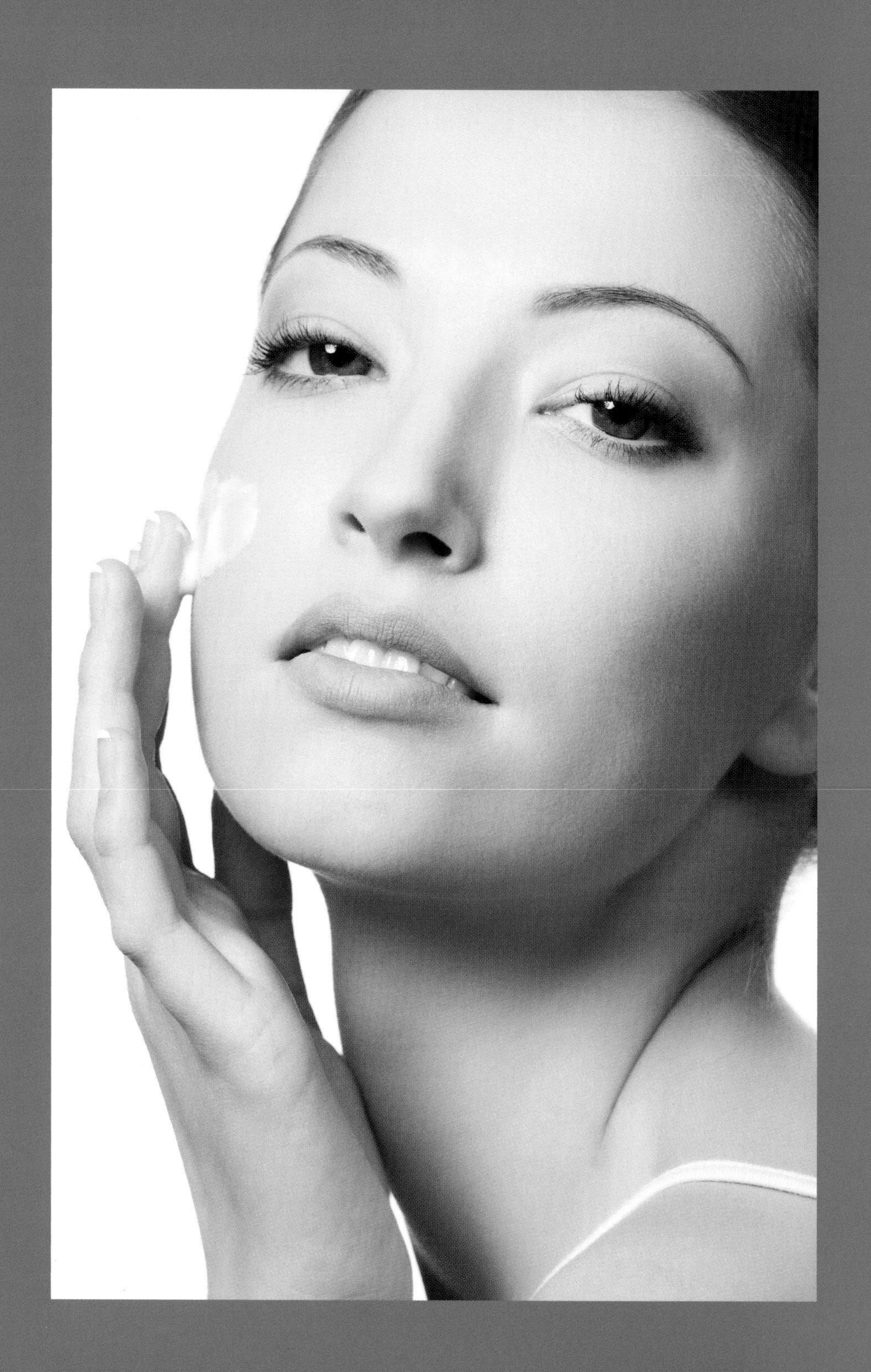

The Basic Regime

Now that we have learned how to diagnose our skin and treat problems, we should examine the way we care for our skin on a daily basis. The following steps are basic for everyone.

Cleanse (detoxify)

Cleansing the skin, day and night, to remove impurities, excess oil, pollution and dirt is the first step. We must start with a clean surface before applying layers of moisture or a barrier. A gentle cleanser which does not strip the acid mantle of the skin is key.

Tone

Toners, as hydrators or PH balancers, are much needed. A toner can tighten the skin's pores, keeping out pollution, bacteria and dirt. Also, the skin will better absorb moisturizer if it is already moist. In Ayurveda, applying oil to wet skin is believed to help it to penetrate more easily.

Moisturize (Nourish)

Moisturizers serve two purposes – to hydrate and to protect the skin. They may also have other ingredients which stimulate, add minerals or disinfect. Using a serum under a rich cream enhances its effects. Since oil does not provide water, and water or serums provide little barrier, a cream is a wonderful mélange of both properties. Layering is most effective as we can tailor each day's regime to our skin's needs based on internal and external conditions. Serum contributes to the barrier function because plump skin cells help guard against water loss and cause the skin's structure to be more dense.

Skincare products are applied in order of weight.

Since light textures penetrate more easily while heavier ones sit on the skin, applying from light to heavy ensures maximum absorption.

Extended Rituals

Exfoliants (detoxify)

Regular exfoliation keeps skin vibrant and young. Frequency and depth will depend on skin type.

Masks

Masks vary in practice and purpose. Though there are an abundance of different kinds on the market, they are usually of these three types:

1. Detoxifying / Drying,
2. Nourishing / Hydrating
3. Exfoliating

Recently, stimulating masks have become more common for promoting circulation, but they are not commonplace yet.

Masks are a great tool for deeply treating the skin. Since clay masks can dry out skin, alternate hydrating masks, or try mixing a purifying clay mask with a nourishing cream mask.

Frequently Asked Questions

Do I really need a toner?

In the past, toners were primarily to clear off the residue from petroleum-based cleansers. Since this is not needed with petroleum-free products, they now are incredibly beneficial for hydration, balancing the skin's PH and contracting pores. Using a cotton pad to apply them, as some people still do, is wasteful of the cotton and the product. Misting is best.

Most toners have specific uses. For example, a chamomile hydrosol is great for calming inflammation, whereas toners with collagen are anti-aging. For those of us who need to prevent breakouts or bacterial infection, an astringent is still of use, but it must not contain drying ingredients like alcohol. Organic peppermint, sage and witch hazel hydrosols are great for disinfecting without stripping, irritating or extracting moisture. Witch hazel is especially good as it also brings down inflammation.

Can I shrink my pores?

While we refer to the pores as "opening" and "closing," they do not so much open and close as soften and contract. Our skin can be in absorption or barrier mode. When wet, it will absorb cream or lotion more easily, and when the skin is hydrated, our pores appear smaller.

Many may think deep absorption can be promoted by simply applying moisturizer to a wet face, but water does not provide the PH balancing that a formulated toner does. Not only do toners promote healthy skin (PH 5.0-5.6: germs do not grow in acidic environments) but they will penetrate more deeply than simple H_2O.

What is the difference between day and night creams?

Day cream:

A day cream is essential for even the most perfect complexions to prevent signs of aging and maintain hydration levels. It is during the day when we are exposed to the elements, pollution and stress. While many people prefer a light day cream, fearing shine and an oily look, a heavier one provides better protection. In drier, harsher climates, a pure oil or barrier cream is advised.

Night cream:

Traditionally night creams are heavier in texture than day creams. At night the skin can absorb and digest larger molecules. While feeding our skin at night can be very effective, many skincare companies no longer advocate this. Their belief is that the skin detoxifies and purges toxins during sleep as the body regenerates. While the elimination of a night moisturizer may be uncomfortable for the first two weeks, the skin will gradually adjust. We can compromise by using a light moisturizer, serum or concentrated liquid ampoule, instead of a heavy cream, to respect this process of detoxification while also nourishing.

I personally believe that the use of night creams depends on the individual. If the skin is severely depleted, night-time nourishment is excellent, especially for those, like acne sufferers, who are afraid of the feeling of oil or heaviness during the day. The other factor is climate. In winter, we often reside in dry, heated environments which take their toll and require us to replenish as much as possible.

For simplicity's sake, I prefer the same day and night moisturizer, but once again, circumstances alter cases.

Why should I get facials?

I love facials. With air travel being the fastest-growing source of greenhouse emissions, and cruise ships producing an average of one hundred thousand liters of sewage per day, an all-natural spa day provides a far more eco-friendly timeout. Facials also tone the skin through stimulation and purification, and are part of any proactive skincare routine.

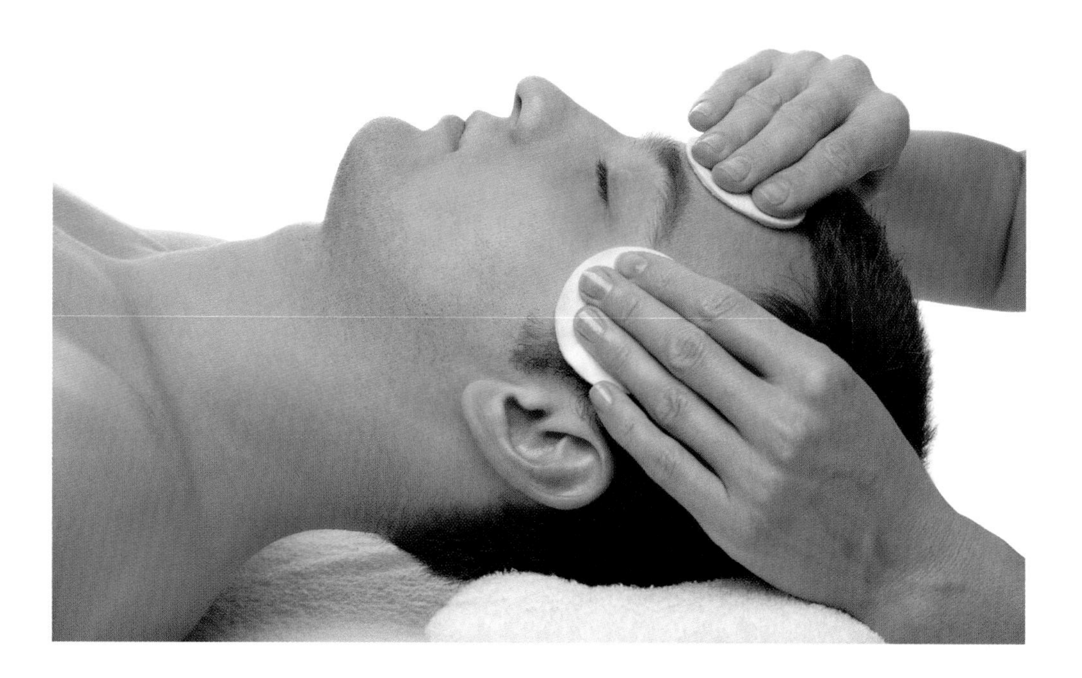

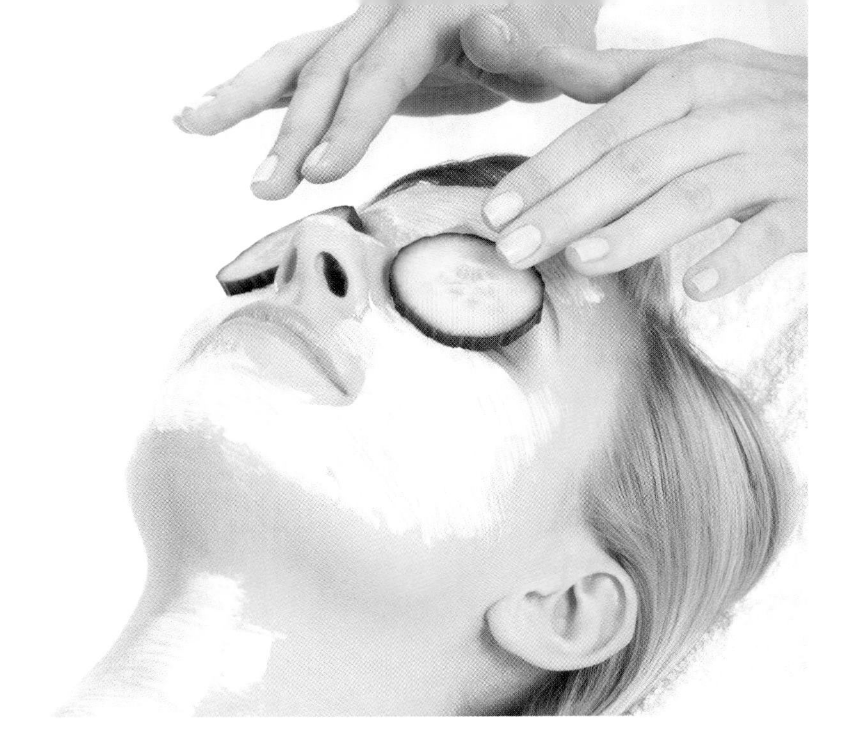

Facials

Detoxify, move and nourish.
A good facial should encompass all three functions:

1. Detoxify your skin and pores
2. Move the blood, lymphatic system and face muscles
3. Nourish and treat the skin

Habitual facials are integral to keeping our skin in balance and clearing it of impurities.

Those who seek simple maintenance will ideally treat their skin every four-to-six weeks. Acne-prone skin may need a treatment every two-to-three weeks for more vigorous pore-cleansing. Those actively combating anti-aging may want weekly treatments geared to specific goals.

The Steps of a Facial

The following are the basic steps in a facial. While some treatments may incorporate body work or different kinds of exfoliation, these are the fundamentals.

Cleanse

Cleansing the skin opens the ritual by providing a blank canvas. Makeup, pollution, excess sebum and skincare residue are cleared away to prevent contamination. This detoxifying step should be gentle, non-stripping and non-disruptive to the skin's acid mantle.

Exfoliate

Exfoliation is an extension of the cleansing process, aimed at clearing away dead cells and congestion. While some treatments may use a granular peel, others will use an AHA, gommage or Sea-salt Microdermabrasion. This helps pore-extraction by unclogging and moisturizing the skin through polishing. At Pure + Simple we do not exfoliate our sensitive clients. We simply apply collagen and oil under the steam to minimize redness during extractions and to prepare the skin for the next process.

Steam

Steam is so beneficial for opening/softening the pores. It is also hydrating because the skin accepts steam at a deeper level. Any essential oils, etc., will also penetrate deeper. Some people with sensitive skin may prefer to skip the steam. Instead of their vetoing the entire step, I suggest you request rosewater pads to be applied to sensitive areas as a barrier. The hydration and warmth will lessen inflammation from extractions.

Extract

A good facial involves thorough extractions. This purging of toxins is vital to prevent stagnation and further enlargement of the pores. Keep in mind, "good extractions" do not mean aggressive extractions; it means purifying the skin in a way that is professional, careful and meticulous.

An experienced esthetician will know where to press on the skin and how much pressure is enough for each condition so as never to scar or bruise. Extractions are something we should not do ourselves because often we are too harsh and determined, causing trauma.

Face Massage

Face, shoulder and scalp massage is not only for relaxation. This part of the facial – the most enjoyable for some! – should stimulate the circulation and the muscles, while draining the lymph system and tissues of excess fluid. In TCM, tuina (acupressure massage) is said to be excellent for stimulating collagen and elastin production. It is also nourishing, and should be done with a natural face oil.

Mask

Masks should be individualized to each person's needs. They can be mixed to personalize them. Example: combining soothing and detoxifying masks for congested, sensitive skin.

Tone, Moisturize and Protect

We must always protect our skin before exposing it to the environment. This is especially true in urban settings. Each facial treatment must end with toning and moisturizing. Of course, these must treat individual needs. At Pure + Simple, we often will exfoliate just before this step (if not done previously) to better enhance the penetration of toners and moisturizers. Sunscreen or mineral makeup is also applied for protection.

Facials as Total Body Experiences

At Pure + Simple, we believe in holistic facial treatments. This encompasses the mind, body and spirit. The emotional and spiritual rejuvenation that these treatments offer also translates into physical results. When the mind is at peace, our bodies become attuned to this state as well.

A facial that also treats the body gives the recipient full-body stimulation as well as total-body relaxation.

Body and Hair Care

Because we absorb so much through our skin, we should be aware of products we use on all parts of our body and our hair.

The skin is our largest organ, yet typically we treat it in sections. Though many of us only moisturize our faces daily, by oiling our bodies and scalps we also boost moisture in our facial skin because it is a single organ.

Oiling, according to Ayurveda is cleansing, and full-body oiling also lubricates our muscles and organs helping to loosen toxins from these areas. For example, oiling our tummies lubricates our intestines and GI tract.

Moistening the body and scalp also helps circulation by keeping the capillaries moist, especially if you use warming oils like sesame and avocado. In particular, those of us with cold hands and feet benefit from oiling them nightly.

Many Ayurvedic remedies for psychological disorders (Vata) involve oiling the scalp. Due to the porousness of hair follicles, the scalp is especially susceptible to deep absorption. This was demonstrated by a study which observed hairless versus hairy mice and found those with hair absorbed two to three times more topically.

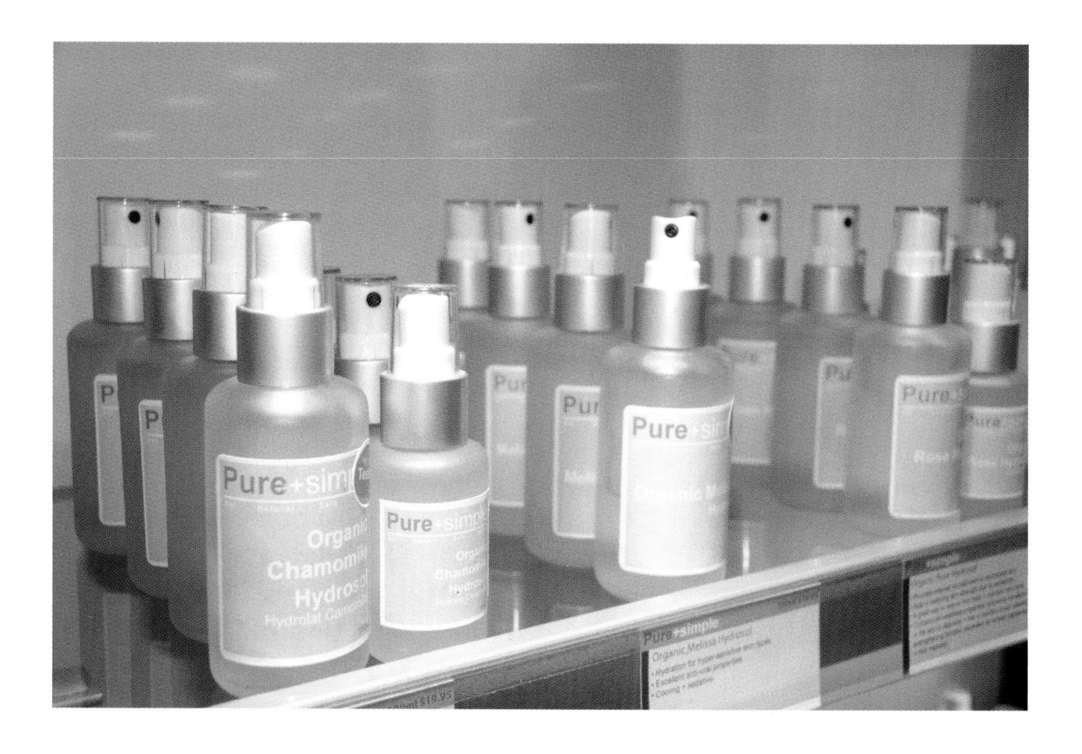

Makeup

Cosmetics have high status in our medicine cabinets. Every woman (and some men) knows how a little makeup can create a huge difference in enhancing and defining our natural features.

But often we overlook what chemicals our makeup contains. We make sure our cleansers are non-stripping, our toners are PH-balancing, and our creams are protective, soothing, non-clogging and moisturizing. We spend hours (and fortunes) finding a regime which best suits our skin's needs and conditions, then we apply heavy liquid foundations, clogging concealers, drying powders and irritating rouges and shadows, undoing all our hard work. Still, not many of us are willing to go makeup free.

There have been many advances in natural cosmetics, resulting in more lines using natural ingredients (though some still contain cornstarch, which is natural, but dehydrates the skin). In the past, these natural brands did not have the staying power or vibrancy of chemical ones, so many professional women opted for practicality over purity. But we no longer need to make this compromise as the invention of mineral makeup has married clean ingredients with modern functionality.

Mineral makeup

My favorite cosmetic find was mineral makeup. When I was going through the acne-era of my life, I struggled to find a way to camouflage my skin without promoting more blemishes. I found mineral cosmetics to be invaluable for helping me through a very self-conscious period of my youth, allowing me to wear foundation without clogging my pores, and providing SPF protection that helped my vulnerable skin after frantic over-peeling.

Mineral Makeup Explained

Mineral cosmetics are composed of one hundred per cent pressed or loose minerals – zinc, titanium, iron, etc. They do not have dyes or perfumes which are known to clog or irritate, and a quality brand will press these mineral powders with wax or oil rather than chemicals. The minerals themselves are beneficial. Zinc (as mentioned in our sun block discussion) is anti-bacterial, anti-inflammatory and is a natural sun protector. Mineral makeup is perfect for rosacea, acne, allergic and aging skin, since it is completely natural and soothes as it purifies.

Mineral Coverage

The first question my mature clients ask is: *Will the powder make me look old?* Despite the best ingredients and benefits, if a product makes us look old, it is going into the garbage.

Pure + Simple mineral powders (and liquids) do not contain drying ingredients, like talc or cornstarch, so they do not cake or go on powdery and flaky. The light-reflecting properties of the minerals actually create a look that brightens, while hiding imperfections.

These minerals provide the complete pigment of this makeup, so chemical dyes are not required as with most other cosmetics. They possess amazing, long-lasting effects and are even water-resistant for up to 40 minutes.

Application

It is easy. Apply evenly with a clean brush or sponge. Apply in layers, adding more opaqueness as desired, and giving equal amounts of sun protection all over the face.

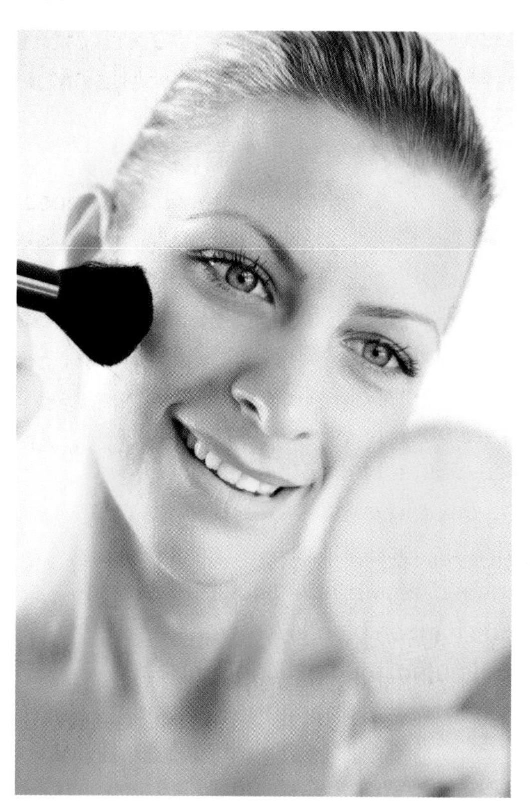

The only trick is that skin must be moist underneath or the powder will not hold properly. Dry on dry skin will not adhere just as liquid foundations slide off oily skin types throughout the day (oil on oil). For very dehydrated skin, I first apply a rich moisturizer or face oil before a mineral powder. Even oily skin with dehydration can use a natural face oil to create a seamless, finished look similar to that of a liquid foundation.

Liquid mineral products are applied like any other liquid foundation.

Makeovers 101

1. Start with a clean base. Camouflaging skin imperfections to even the tone will make an immediate difference. When blocking redness, blemishes, dark spots and circles, the features become more prominent. For example, lessening redness will make the colour of the eyes more brilliant. Sometimes full foundation is not necessary, a little dab of concealer will do the trick; however, using a mineral base is beneficial for protecting the skin. If you do want an all-over foundation, colour-match it to the skin on your neck so you won't look like you are wearing a mask. If your neck and face are very different in colour, pick an in-between shade to blend and even this out.

2. Tend to your brows. Eyebrows are my favourite part of a makeover, and one of our most influential features. Darkening them will give the face more definition, while lightening them softens it. Always keep in mind that the brows frame the eyes. If they are too thick or dark they will overpower and take attention from the beauty of the eyes. If they are too light the complexion will look washed out. Lifting the arch of the brows is something to consider with mature skin, to increase the look of youthfulness. If you are unsure of how to groom them, consult an esthetician.

3. Contour to shape the face. As a woman of Asian decent, I have a flat nose and shallow features. While shallow features are very beautiful, they can look swollen and shapeless. For this reason, I often contour my nose and cheekbones (especially on puffy-face days). Remember that dark colour creates shadows and pushes in, while light colour highlights and pushes out. I will put dark contour on the sides of my nose and light on the tip of it. I will also camouflage turkey neck with dark contour under the jaw line and down the front of the throat. Of course, we must always blend for a natural, flawless look.

4. Give yourself some colour. Using a blush or bronzer will create a healthy glow. After using a foundation, you may look unnatural without blush because you have blocked out your natural cheek color. I have noticed, when doing television segments without heavy blush, that I looked more masculine and flat-faced. Because TV blanches us out, more colour than usual is needed, amplifying what we should do day-to-day. When applying blush, start from the temples and blend down into the cheeks and along the cheekbone to contour and chisel the face. Applying soft, circular colour only on the apples of the cheeks will emphasize that area and soften the face.

5. Moisten the lips. Whatever else you do, always keep your lips moist. Even if you wear a matte lipstick to give more attention to the eyes, do not use products which suck out moisture. Chapped lips are never in style. Glosses will create a pouty, full-lipped look while matte lipsticks flatten. Whichever you choose, the best products treat the lips while making you look great.

6. Suit your lifestyle. Always choose cosmetics which are appropriate to the way you live. If you do not have time to reapply throughout the day, choose colours with less contrast to avoid the look of fading and colour-bleeding. If you work in a professional environment, choose makeup which communicates your work persona. Light pastels can be youthful and soft, while darker colours and contrasting makeup are more dramatic. Do not choose what is in vogue, but what suits your colouring. Generally, dark, stark makeup is most easily carried off by people with contrast in their natural coloring. Dark-haired, fair-skinned people can wear wine reds and chocolate browns. Lighter, softer colors (and textures) are most suitable for people with little natural contrast. Of course, this is a general rule which can be broken to achieve a specific look.

These are simple guidelines. Always use what makes you feel beautiful, comfortable and attractive.

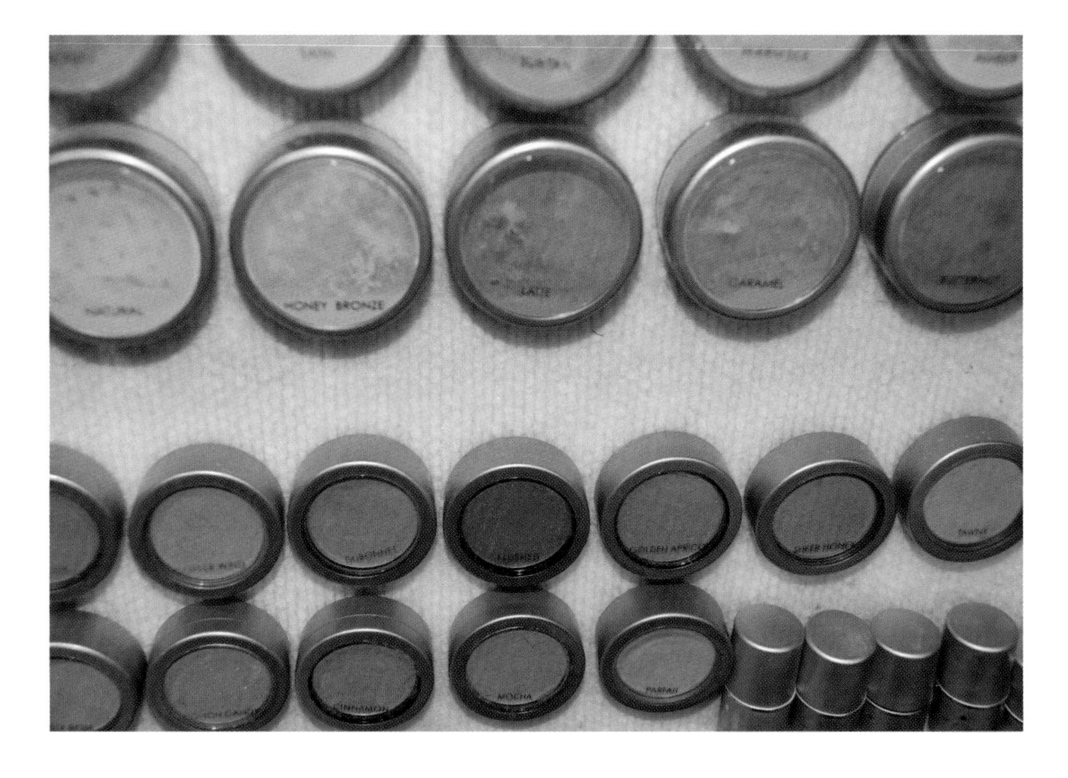

Beauty 2.0

I hope, after reading this book, you will share my passion for natural skincare as it inspires a new concept of beauty. In this modern age, we must change our old definition, to one which fits the world we live in and benefits our society.

Beauty as a Feeling

To me, beauty is a feeling. While beauty means different things to different people, I describe it as health because it radiates vibrancy and fullness. When we see beauty, we experience awe.

I remember overhearing a conversation about the Northern Lights in my doctor's office. The receptionist was talking to one of the other patients about once having seen them and she said it was the most beautiful experience she had ever had. She continued to say that now, whenever she was depressed, she remembered that vision and would feel her spirits lift.

Whether found in a person, place or an object, beauty is to me something weighted with a sense of elation, happiness, contentedness, purpose in living. When we feel beautiful, we feel grounded and confident enough to face the world with happiness and pride. Many of us are so desperate for this feeling of beauty that we will undertake dangerous procedures to possess it. Such practices are never really effective in the long-term because they are based on an unhealthy idea of beauty.

Beauty as a Mirror for Our Values

Beauty has always been a reflection of cultural norms and values. It is symbolic of who we want to be and what we find admirable.

In the Agrarian Age, beauty was very much about youth and fertility. Robustness and stamina were prized because they meant the ability to procreate and to contribute to the community's survival. Traces of this view still exist as a biological predisposition. As civilization progressed, humans began to treasure full-bodied women who showed no aptitude for manual work, as a reflection of leisure-class status. These divergent views show us how much beauty is about a desired lifestyle rather than about the physical magnetism of an ideal.

With the coming of the industrial age, humans accepted a more manufactured idea of beauty. The productivity of standard rules for our legal system, our workplace, our consumer goods, was reflected in a standardized view of beauty. It became defined as mannequin-esque facial features along with sculpted, cookie-cutter bodies. We are still very much in this era, which is why many of us wish for more chiseled features, longer legs and tinier waists to match our society's conventional tastes.

But there are signs that we are now entering a more knowledge-focused age, in which we must change our definition of beauty just as we are changing our values. With new issues, new threats to our survival and new technology, we must align our views of what is attractive and desirable to reflect this shift in thinking.

Beauty must become an embodiment of wisdom, consciousness and self-empowerment. This would support a move toward the less excessive, less uncompromising and more inclusive. This is why I hope this book becomes a useful part of how we can better live our lives. It not only promotes clear skin and healthy bodies, but self-respect and a positive promotion of beauty.

Be Part of the Change

Change must come from us first. Often we think society must do the changing, while forgetting that collectively we *are* society. It is our individual responsibility to help change general beliefs, instead of allowing ourselves to be sabotaged by them.

This understanding came to me while I was listening to CBC's Radio One. There was a discussion about pornography's influence on sex roles in our society and the speaker was the author of a book which explored this subject. He was stressing how much the sex industry has shaped what we think of as "sexy" because so many young people look to internet pornography as a guide to sexual dynamics. He described these dynamics as misogynistic and he stated he thought this would have long-term repercussions on the self-image of women. But more interesting, he introduced the finding that some women believed pornography to be empowering as it asserted female desirability. He thought this reflected the dysfunction of female roles in our society as he stated: "Any woman knows beauty is fleeting in our society as it is considered synonymous with youth. If a woman cannot sustain sexual attractiveness through maturity, the idea of power through sex is a fallacy."

This spurred a revelation for me: it is often women who accept these images and promote them to each other. Yet, when dominated by this youthful, pornographic image, we can never feel beautiful in middle age. It is up to us to change this social norm to a more positive one. Because I do not believe beauty is about being perfectly proportioned, I have found women highly attractive because of the power in their voices; I have found men attractive because of the beauty of their intentions, and I have found myself most beautiful when I am living my life in a holistic way.

So, I hope this book not only offers the tools and knowledge to upkeep our bodies, but also an understanding of how subtle, healthy practices can yield powerful and positive outcomes.

I believe that beauty, as an intangible feeling of being comfortable in our own skins, affects how we conduct ourselves. If we feel ugly or out of balance, we may not be in the right headspace to be open-minded, unselfish and positive. A change in the definition of beauty is a change is the way we view our world. We must commit ourselves to this responsibility. I see people gravitating towards this already. It is not my movement, but a natural change that already resonates with many people. Pure + Simple has been successful not only because natural skincare is in vogue, but because, finally, there is a company that aligns itself with the way many people now want to live.

I believe the Pure + Simple concept is not just a way to groom ourselves, but a lifestyle. This new cultural phenomenon is about respect for others, the environment and ourselves. It is about a world where ideas will be more valuable than goods, and where status will come through societal contribution, not an accumulation of wealth. It is not a change that I alone want, but a change that must happen if we are going to ensure the healthiness of our communities.

The future is ambiguous, but I have faith that we will enter into an age of consciousness and flexibility, with the old, rigid norms becoming outdated and inapplicable. Beauty, as superficial as people may think it to be, is central to this change because beauty is really about embodying what we value.

Beauty 2.0 – I am excited for the future.

Index

Endnotes

P. 19 Natural Skincare Definition – Wallace, B. (2007). Setting the Standard for natural beauty care. *Delicious Living*, 23(3), 16.

P. 22 We absorb everything on our skin – Vance, J. (1999). *Beauty to Die For.* New York: toExcel.

P. 24 Hormones in drinking water: the effect on our bodies and marine species –

Pindera, L. (2007, December 5) *Plastics.* The Current. Toronto: Canadian Broadcasting Corporation.

P. 29-30 Functions of the skin (Detoxification, Regulating Body Temperature, Protection) – Pulgliese, P. T. (1999). *Skin, Sex and Longevity.* Bernville, PA: TPG.

P. 30-31 Absorption – Vance, J. (1999). *Beauty to Die For.* New York: toExcel.

P. 37 Gender and Skin Texture – Pugliese, P. T. (2001). *Physiology of the Skin II.* Carol Stream: Allured Publishing Corporation.

P. 41 Ayurveda: Definition – Svoboda, R.E. (1988). *Prakriti.* Bellingham: Sadhana Publications.

P. 48 Menstruation and Dosha predominance – Svoboda, R.E. (2000). *Ayurveda for Women.* Rochester: Healing Arts Press.

P. 49-50 Which Doshas are prominent in each stage of life – Svoboda, R.E. (2000). *Ayurveda for Women.* Rochester: Healing Arts Press.

P. 57 Ayurveda and Face Mapping – Raichur, P. (1997). *Absolute Beauty.* New York: Harper Collins Publishers.

P. 59-60 Parts of the Face in Relationship to the Internal Organs – Kushi, M. (1983). *Your Face Never Lies.* USA: Avery.

P. 61 Internal Organs and how they are expressed – American Foundation of Traditional Chinese Medicine. (1997). *Chinese Medicine.* London: Carlton Books.

P. 61 Zang and Fu Organs – American Foundation of Traditional Chinese Medicine. (1997). *Chinese Medicine.* London: Carlton Books.

P. 67-68 Petroleum and its harmful effects on the internal body – Vance, J. (1999). *Beauty to Die For.* New York: toExcel.

P. 69 SLS and its harmful effects on the internal body – Vance, J. (1999). *Beauty to Die For.* New York: toExcel.

P. 70-71 The damage of other harmful chemicals – Vance, J. (1999). *Beauty to Die For.* New York: toExcel.

P. 75 Adrenals and Stress – Thompson, D. (2005). *The Ayurvedic Diet.* New Delhi: New Age Books.

P. 77 Stress and Fat due to Cortisol – Schuba, V. (2001). *Combatting Cellulite.* Oxford: Meyer & Meyer.

P. 87 Drinking Charged Water to Hydrate – Wolfe, D. (2007). *Eating for Beauty.* San Diego: Sun Food Publishing.

P. 91 – Pollution and Exhaust Fumes can create Skin Damage – Maes, D. (2004) *The Ins and Outs of Skin Protection Technology.* Society of Cosmetic Chemists Ontario Chapter Presents Healthy Skin, Toronto, Ontario.

P. 101 Puffy eyes and Kapha – Raichur, P. (1997). *Absolute Beauty.* New York: Harper Collins Publishers.

P. 101 Causes of Cholesterol Deposits – Pirello, C. (2001). *Glow*. New York: HP Books

P. 102 Lips and their relation to the Digestive Organs – Lad, V. (1985). *The Science of Self-Healing*. Wilmot: Lotus Press.

P. 117-119 Types of Acne – Acne.org. (2008). *What is acne?* http://www.acne.org/whatisacne.html

P. 120 The Aggressiveness of Accutane – Adderly, B., Dubrow, T. (2003). *The Acne Cure*. New York: Warner Books.

P. 120 Psychiatric side effects of Accutane – Accutane Suicide Help Line. (2008). *Homepage*. http://www.accutane-suicide-help.com

P. 127 The Four Faces of Rosacea – Rosacea.org. (2007). *Coping with Rosacea*. http://www.rosacea.org/patients/materials/coping/stages.php

P. 129 Characteristics of Eczema – Orton, C. (1986). *Eczema*. Bungay: Richard Clay Ltd.

P. 132 The Darkeness Explained – Pugliese, P. T. (2001). *Physiology of the Skin II*. Carol Stream: Allured Publishing Corporation.

Potter, N. (2007, October). *Understanding Pigmentation*. The Medical, Spa and Esthetics Conference, Toronto, Ontario.

P. 133 Pigmentation caused by Vata in the Blood – Lad, V., (2002). *Textbook of Ayurveda* Albuquerque: Ayurvedic Press.

P. 138 Sugar and Freckles – Pirello, C. (2001). *Glow*. New York: HP Books.

P. 139 Ayurveda and Menopause – Svoboda, R.E. (2000). *Ayurveda for Women*. Rochester: Healing Arts Press.

P. 142 Beans and Soy as Elastase Inhibitors – Pugliese, P. T. (2001). *Physiology of the Skin II*. Carol Stream: Allured Publishing Corporation.

P. 142 The effect of Free radicals and Lipofuscin – Pugliese, P. T. (2001). *Physiology of the Skin II*. Carol Stream: Allured Publishing Corporation.

P. 143 Description and behaviors of specific Free Radicals – Pugliese, P. T. (2001). *Physiology of the Skin II*. Carol Stream: Allured Publishing Corporation.

P. 146 The Damage of Deep Peels – Muller, M. (2006). Facial Reflexology. Rochester: Healing Arts Press.

P. 147 Descriptions of IPL and Lasers – Piantino, M. (2007, October). *Understanding Photo Dynamic Therapy, IPL/VPL, LED and Laser Technology*. The Medical, Spa and Esthetics Conference, Toronto, Ontario.

P. 162 Study of Hairless Versus Hairy Mice and Absorption – Vance, J. (1999). *Beauty to Die For*. New York: toExcel.

References

Accutane Suicide Help Line. (2008). Homepage. Retrieved from: http://www.accutane-suicide-help.com

Acne.org. (2008). *What is acne? Retrieved from*: http://www.acne.org/whatisacne.html

Adderly, B., Dubrow, T. (2003). *The Acne Cure*. New York: Warner Books.

American Foundation of Traditional Chinese Medicine. (1997). *Chinese Medicine*. London: Carlton Books.

Kushi, M. (1983). *Your Face Never Lies*. USA: Avery.

Lad, V. (1985). *The Science of Self-Healing*. Wilmot: Lotus Press.

Lad, V., (2002). *Textbook of Ayurveda* Albuquerque: Ayurvedic Press.

Maes, D. (2004) *The Ins and Outs of Skin Protection Technology*. Society of Cosmetic Chemists Ontario Chapter Presents Healthy Skin, Toronto, Ontario.

Muller, M. (2006). *Facial Reflexology*. Rochester: Healing Arts Press.

Orton, C. (1986). *Eczema*. Bungay: Richard Clay Ltd.

Piantino, M. (2007, October). *Understanding Photo Dynamic Therapy, IPL/VPL, LED and Laser Technology*. The Medical, Spa and Esthetics Conference, Toronto, Ontario.

Pindera, L. (2007, December 5) *Plastics*. The Current. Toronto: Canadian Broadcasting Corporation.

Pirello, C. (2001). *Glow*. New York: HP Books.

Potter, N. (2007, October). *Understanding Pigmentation*. The Medical, Spa and Esthetics Conference, Toronto, Ontario.

Pugliese, P. T. (2001). *Physiology of the Skin II*. Carol Stream, IL: Allured Publishing Corporation.

Pulgliese, P. T. (1999). *Skin, Sex and Longevity*. Bernville, PA: TPG.

Raichur, P. (1997). *Absolute Beauty*. New York: HarperCollins Publishers.

Rosacea.org. (2007). *Coping with Rosacea*. Retrieved from http://www.rosacea.org/patients/materials/coping/stages.php

Schuba, V. (2001). *Combatting Cellulite*. Oxford: Meyer & Meyer.

Svoboda, R.E. (1988). *Prakriti*. Bellingham, WA: Sadhana Publications.

Svoboda, R.E. (2000). *Ayurveda for Women*. Rochester: Healing Arts Press.

Thompson, D. (2005). *The Ayurvedic Diet*. New Delhi: New Age Books.

Vance, J. (1999). *Beauty to Die For*. New York: toExcel.

Wallace, B. (2007). Setting the Standard for natural beauty care. *Delicious Living*, 23(3), 16.

Wolfe, D. (2007). *Eating for Beauty*. San Diego: Sun Food Publishing.

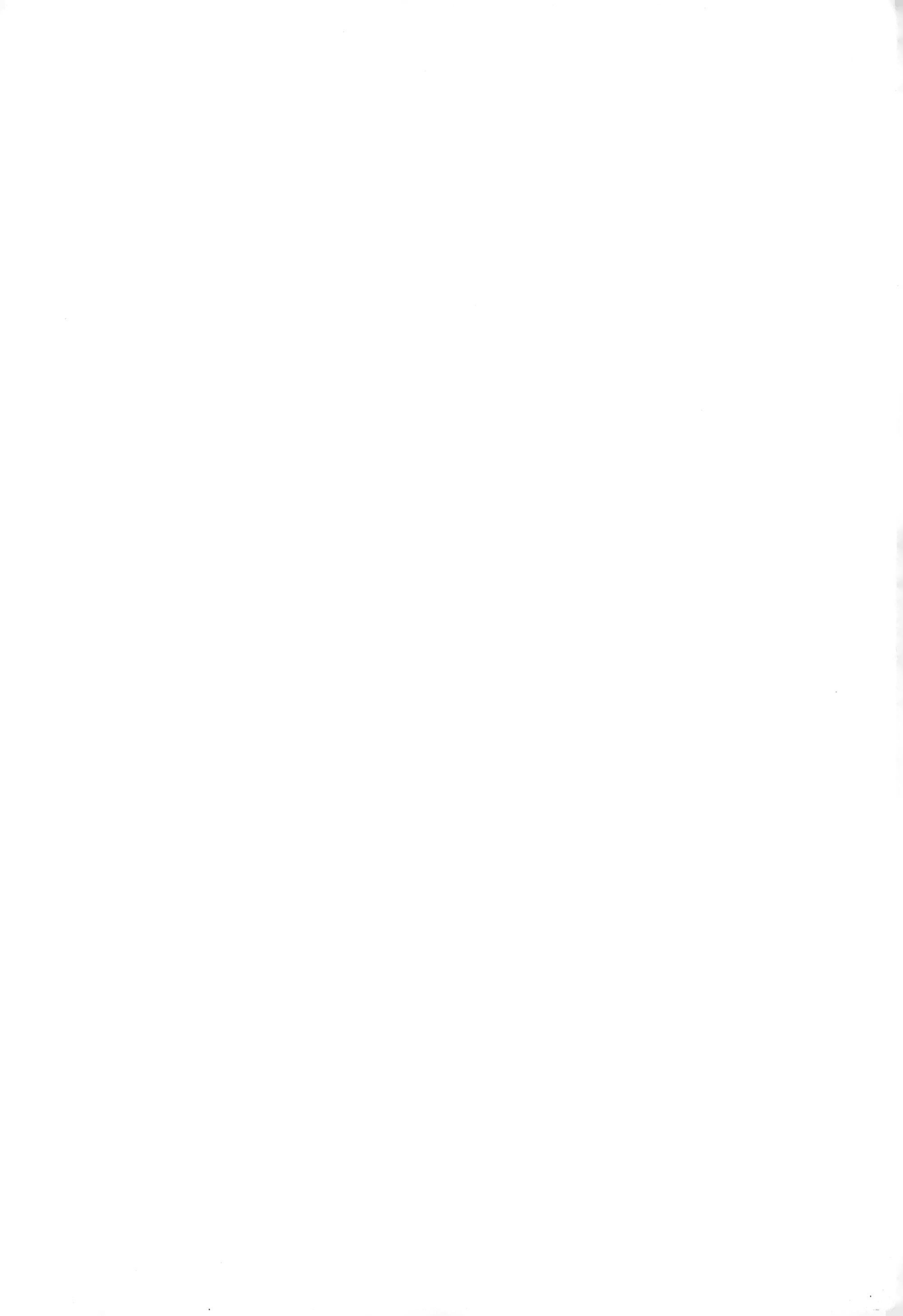